Premenstrual Dysphorias

Myths and Realities

Premenstrual Dysphorias

Myths and Realities

Edited by

Judith H. Gold, M.D., F.R.C.P.C.
Member, American Psychiatric Association Task Force for DSM-IV
Chairperson, DSM-IV Work Group on Late Luteal Phase
Dysphoric Disorder
Halifax, Nova Scotia, Canada

Sally K. Severino, M.D.
Associate Professor of Clinical Psychiatry
New York Hospital–Cornell Medical Center, Westchester Division
White Plains, New York

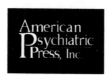

American Psychiatric Press, Inc.

Washington, DC
London, England

Copyright © 1994 American Psychiatric Press, Inc.
ALL RIGHTS RESERVED
Manufactured in the United States of America on acid-free paper
97 96 95 94   4 3 2 1
First Edition

American Psychiatric Press, Inc.
1400 K Street, N.W., Washington, DC   20005

Library of Congress Cataloging-in-Publication Data
Premenstrual dysphorias : myths and realities / editors, Judith H.
  Gold, Sally K. Severino. — 1st ed.
     p.   cm.
  Prepared by the DSM-IV Work Group on Late Luteal Phase Dysphoric
Disorder.
  Includes bibliographical references and index.
  ISBN 0-88048-666-X
  1. Premenstrual syndrome.   2. Premenstrual syndrome—
classification.   3. Premenstrual syndrome—Social aspects.
I. Gold, Judith H., 1941–   . II. Severino, Sally K.   III. American
Psychiatric Association.   DSM-IV Work Group on Late Luteal Phase
Dysphoric Disorder.
  [DNLM: 1. Premenstrual Syndrome—classification.   2. Premenstrual
Syndrome—psychology.   3. Premenstrual Syndrome—diagnosis.
4. Luteal Phase—psychology.   5. Mental Disorders—classification.
6. Mental Disorders—diagnosis.   7. Knowledge, Attitudes, Practice.
WP 560 P925 1994]
RG165.P69 1994
618.1'72—dc20
DNLM/DLC
for Library of Congress   93-47479
                                                                      CIP

British Library Cataloguing in Publication Data
A CIP record is available from the British Library.

To our husbands,
who have encouraged us to understand
the nature of women's struggles.

❧ Contents ❧

I
Empirical Issues

∂ Contributors ℰ

Alice J. Dan, Ph.D.
Professor, College of Nursing, and Director, Center for Research on Women and Gender, University of Illinois at Chicago, Chicago, Illinois

*Jean Endicott, Ph.D.
Professor of Clinical Psychology in Psychiatry, Columbia University College of Physicians and Surgeons, New York State Psychiatric Institute, New York, New York

Allen Frances, M.D.
Chairperson, American Psychiatric Association Task Force for DSM-IV; Professor and Chairman of Psychiatry, Duke University Medical Center, Durham, North Carolina

*Ellen Frank, Ph.D.
Associate Professor of Psychiatry and Psychology, Western Psychiatric Institute and Clinic, Pittsburgh, Pennsylvania

*Judith H. Gold, M.D., F.R.C.P.C.
Member, American Psychiatric Association Task Force for DSM-IV; Chairperson, DSM-IV Work Group on Late Luteal Phase Dysphoric Disorder, Halifax, Nova Scotia, Canada

Bryna Harwood, B.A.
Medical Student, The University of Chicago, School of Medicine, Chicago, Illinois

---

*Member, American Psychiatric Association DSM-IV Work Group on Late Luteal Phase Dysphoric Disorder.

Stephen W. Hurt, Ph.D.
Associate Professor of Clinical Psychology in Psychiatry, New York Hospital–Cornell Medical Center, Westchester Division, White Plains, New York

Lisa Monagle, Ph.D., C.N.M.
Department of Social and Preventive Medicine, State University of New York at Buffalo, Buffalo, New York

Mary Brown Parlee, Ph.D.
Professor of Psychology, The Graduate School and University Center, City University of New York Graduate Center, New York, New York

*
Barbara L. Parry, M.D.
Associate Professor of Psychiatry, University of California, San Diego, La Jolla, California

Teri B. Pearlstein, M.D.
Clinical Assistant Professor of Psychiatry, Western Psychiatric Institute and Clinic, University of Pittsburgh, Pittsburgh, Pennsylvania

Renee Rhodes, B.A.
Senior Research Associate, Western Psychiatric Institute and Clinic, University of Pittsburgh, Pittsburgh, Pennsylvania

Ana Rivera-Tovar, Ph.D.
Senior Clinician, Western Psychiatric Institute and Clinic, University of Pittsburgh, Pittsburgh, Pennsylvania

Paula P. Schnurr, Ph.D.
Research Associate Professor of Psychiatry, Dartmouth Medical School, National Center for Posttraumatic Stress Disorder, Veterans Administration Medical and Regional Office Center, White River Junction, Vermont

*Sally K. Severino, M.D.
Associate Professor of Clinical Psychiatry, New York Hospital–
Cornell Medical Center, Westchester Division, White Plains,
New York

*Nada L. Stotland, M.D.
Associate Professor of Clinical Psychiatry and Obstetrics and Gynecology, The University of Chicago, Chicago, Illinois

Anna L. Stout, Ph.D.
Associate Clinical Professor, Division of Medical Psychology, De-
partments of Psychiatry and Obstetrics and Gynecology, Duke
University Medical Center, Durham, North Carolina

♫ Foreword ♫

This book culminates the efforts of the DSM-IV Work Group on Late Luteal Phase Dysphoric Disorder (LLPDD) to determine the most appropriate placement (if any) of this proposed new category in the diagnostic manual. In the preparation of DSM-III-R, this question was the subject of a bitter and unfortunate controversy between those who were convinced that LLPDD should be included as an official category in the main body of the classification and those who were equally convinced that it should not be included anywhere in the manual. As is true of most bitter controversies, both positions were supported by plausible (and even compelling) arguments. And, of course, few were happy with the eventual compromise that placed the criteria set in an appendix for Proposed Diagnostic Categories Needing Further Study—a limbo that offered neither official recognition nor official banishment.*

In preparing DSM-IV, we have placed our greatest emphasis on the need for a systematic review of the available empirical data as a guide for all discussion and decision making. The DSM-IV Work Group on LLPDD conducted an extremely thorough review that, in modified and much expanded form, is the book you are about to read. This is a very useful document that far transcends the particular purpose that stimulated its development. The balance of arguments for and against the placement of LLPDD in DSM-IV is certainly much better informed than was possible for DSM-III-R, but the question remains no less difficult to decide. More important than the fate of LLPDD in DSM-IV is the light shed by the work group's effort on what is known, and what is not known, about the proposed diagnosis. However we classify LLPDD, or choose not to

---

Editors' note: Please see the Appendix to this book for the DSM-IV terminology.

classify it, this book will be of great help to clinicians, to researchers, to those interested in how contextual factors influence what is considered health and disorder, and, finally and most important, to those women whose lives can be improved by more specific diagnosis and treatment.

Allen Frances, M.D.

ℛ Acknowledgments ℛ

We would like to thank the many people who have helped us prepare this manuscript. We are especially grateful to our colleagues Orli Avi-Yonah, Ph.D., Stephen Hurt, Ph.D., Margaret Moline, Ph.D., and Paula Schnurr, Ph.D., who have contributed many hours helping us clarify our conceptualization of premenstrual dysphoria.

The librarians at the New York Hospital–Cornell Medical Center, Westchester Division—Marcia Miller, Director; Pamela Quinn; and Stephanie Kopelson—have graciously collected the extensive bibliography we have reviewed.

We owe special gratitude to Danika Kapuschansky, whose excellent computer and graphic art support brought this manuscript to fruition.

ℒ Introduction ℛ

This book describes the issues surrounding the concept of premenstrual dysphoria, including both 1) empirical issues related to the state of the art of the literature and methodological problems and 2) sociocultural issues, including early medical approaches to menstruation and myths about menstruation. It presents the current reality of late luteal phase dysphoric disorder (LLPDD) as viewed by the DSM-IV Work Group on LLPDD in conjunction with the Work Group Advisers. Some chapters (Chapters 1, 3, 5, and 8) were written as part of the DSM-IV process and present a review of the literature through 1991. The other chapters broaden the discussion and include literature published through 1992. The book concludes with recommendations for the future.

Because the symptoms of LLPDD are not specific for the disorder, it is important to rule out all other possible diagnoses as well as to establish a woman's monthly symptom profile in the process of arriving at a definitive diagnosis. This is the art and science of medicine. Disorders are carefully defined according to criteria that are explicitly stated and rigorously applied. At times, of course, more than one disorder can occur simultaneously in the same individual. The problem then for the clinician is to determine what is causing each symptom and how to treat each. For the researcher, the problem is to separate symptoms into their respective disorders to ensure proper investigation of the etiology of the disease and to allow for replication at another time.

This book begins with Dr. Endicott's examination, in Chapter 1, of this process as it relates to LLPDD. The occurrence of other mental and physical disorders together with LLPDD symptoms confounds investigation if they are not considered carefully in each individual case. Dr. Schnurr and her colleagues further describe the difficulties of this process in Chapter 2 by discussing particular methodological issues in the diagnosis of LLPDD, with emphasis on the problem of differentiating women with LLPDD from women without LLPDD in terms of symptom severity, demographic characteristics, and psychiatric history. In general, in medicine we have not found exact ways of measuring the severity of complaints and rely on the person's own perception of the symptoms. This is an important issue for LLPDD, because the diagnosis is based on the woman's daily ratings of her symptoms.

In Chapter 3, Dr. Parry explains the findings from her review of the biological literature conducted for the LLPDD work group. Studies are being reported with increasing frequency since the diagnosis of LLPDD was first placed in the Appendix for conditions needing further study in DSM-III-R in 1987. Dr. Parry outlines the findings through 1991, suggesting that future research should focus on the serotonergic axis.

Dr. Severino further elaborates on this hypothesis in Chapter 4 by extending the review of literature beyond LLPDD to the relationship of the serotonergic system with other diagnoses. She concludes that the serotonergic system seems to be related to the regulation of affects that are present in many different disorders, including LLPDD. In Chapter 5, Dr. Frank, a work group member, and her colleagues review the treatment literature pertaining to premenstrual syndrome (PMS) and LLPDD. Several different treatments have been effective in relieving various premenstrual symptoms, and a few have been promising for LLPDD in some small new studies. The interrelationships of the findings discussed in Chapters 3, 4, and 5 are fascinating and point to the urgent need for synthesis of their meaning through greater research efforts, as well as funding in the area of studies of premenstrual dysphoria. Dr. Parlee, in her discussion of the work group's literature review in Chapter 6, delineates some of the methodological problems in synthesizing the data and suggests a statistical analysis that may clarify certain issues.

The second section of the book focuses on the sociocultural issues that affect both the research into LLPDD and people's beliefs and perceptions about the effects of menstruation on a woman's functioning. In Chapter 7, Dr. Gold describes early medical approaches to menstruation and the research and treatments engendered by these views. Dr. Stotland and Ms. Harwood's discussion in Chapter 8 of the controversies regarding the formalization of a mental disorder related to menses is followed by a discussion of sociocultural influences on the experience of perimenstrual symptoms by Drs. Dan and Monagle in Chapter 9. Dr Severino then provides a commentary on myths and their role in relation to LLPDD in Chapter 10.

In this book, we attempt to present a full discussion of the issues related to the concept of premenstrual dysphoria. Medicine as a field has only lately begun to consider sex differences in research into diseases and their etiologies and treatments. Traditionally, subjects of studies have been men. We discuss how women's monthly cycles have been the focus of so many beliefs over the centuries and why finally examining the scientific basis behind these beliefs is very important. We look at both the biochemical and social aspects of the menstrual cycle. We suggest that PMS and LLPDD be viewed as conditions needing further study that provide a scientific model for conceptualizing the end result of a complicated interaction of biological, psychological, socioeconomic, and cultural forces.

Judith H. Gold, M.D., F.R.C.P.C.

I

Empirical Issues

❧ 1 ❧

Differential Diagnoses and Comorbidity

Jean Endicott, Ph.D.

DSM-III and DSM-III-R and DSM-IV [are] part of the movement toward reliable categorization and measurement. . . . They emphasize clarity and reliability, but sacrifice validity and the whole person.

Hartmann 1992, p. 1139

As with any disorder, once diagnostic criteria are proposed for late luteal phase dysphoric disorder (LLPDD), the first questions to be addressed should be: Can clinicians identify individuals who meet the proposed criteria, and what are the major differential diagnostic issues encountered? Of related importance is the likelihood of concurrent and lifetime comorbidity of a newly defined disorder with other disorders. In addition, as is the case with most medical conditions, some of the clinical features included in the criteria for LLPDD, a disorder characterized by severe premenstrual dysphoric mood and behavioral changes in DSM-III-R (American Psychiatric Association 1987), are shared by other disorders. These clinical features may also be present in other conditions that are not characterized by a level of severity and associated impairment that warrant their consideration as a disorder (e.g., premenstrual changes or syndromes).

Three factors are of major importance for the differential diagnosis of LLPDD: 1) the timing of the appearance (late luteal phase) and disappearance (follicular phase) of a constellation of clinical features, 2) evidence that the clinical features are associated with clinically significant impairment of work, usual social activities, or relationships with others, and 3) evidence that the disturbance is not merely an exacerbation of the symptoms of another disorder. As is the case with most disorders in DSM-III-R, there are no explicit guidelines regarding how these clinical decisions are to be made.

Literature Review

Although the criteria for LLPDD were proposed in 1987, the time lag between their introduction and publication of the results of studies in which the criteria were applied has limited the number of reports relevant to the issues considered in this chapter. The focus here is primarily on studies in which the proposed criteria for LLPDD were applied in clinical and research settings to women who were seeking evaluation and treatment for self-described severe premenstrual problems. Studies whose primary focus has been on determining the best ways to document or calculate the severity of premenstrual and postmenstrual changes in symptoms (e.g., the percent change, effect size, and spectral or trend analysis methods) are discussed elsewhere (see Chapter 2). Although such studies are of both value and methodological interest (Hurt et al. 1992; Magos et al. 1986; Schnurr 1989; Severino et al. 1989; Watkins et al. 1989), for the most part they have not addressed the differential diagnostic issue of severity, in terms of either what constitutes "serious interference" (DSM-III-R, p. 369) or how to differentiate LLPDD that is superimposed on another disorder from other ongoing disorders that are exacerbated during the late luteal phase of the menstrual cycle. Other studies of severe premenstrual problems are not included in the literature review in this chapter because their authors did not relate the measures used to determine severity to the criteria for LLPDD.

The articles listed in Table 1–1 indicate that it is possible for clinicians to identify groups of women who meet the criteria for LLPDD and who do not have any (other) current DSM-III-R Axis I or II disorders. In several of these studies, the authors identified women with other relatively mild conditions who met the criteria for superimposed LLPDD as well (i.e., they had distinct and severe symptoms that were present during the late luteal phase and absent during the follicular phase of the menstrual cycle).

Although, as illustrated by these articles, it is possible to identify women who meet only the LLPDD criteria, women who seek treatment for premenstrual problems are often found to have concurrent mental or other medical conditions that may account for many, if not all, of the "premenstrual" complaints. The most fre-

Table 1–1. Clinical application of the DSM-III-R criteria for late luteal phase dysphoric disorder (LLPDD)

Reference	N subjects	Comments
Rausch et al. 1988	16	Met DSM-III-R criteria for LLPDD
Harrison et al. 1989a	11	Met DSM-III-R criteria for LLPDD
Harrison et al. 1989b	86	Met criteria for LLPDD with no other Axis I or II disorder
	54	Met criteria for LLPDD and also had a relatively mild current anxiety or affective disorder, substance abuse disorder, or personality disorder
Harrison et al. 1989c	14	Sought treatment for severe premenstrual dysphoric changes; diagnosed as meeting criteria for LLPDD with no current Axis I or II disorder
Parry et al. 1989	6	Selected with LLPDD
Harrison et al. 1990	30	Met criteria for LLPDD with no other Axis I or II disorder
Pearlstein et al. 1990	78	Met criteria for LLPDD with no Axis I diagnosis
Stone et al. 1990	50	Met criteria for LLPDD with no Axis I disorder
	20	Met criteria for LLPDD but also had an Axis I disorder

quent conditions requiring differential diagnostic attention are indicated in Tables 1–2, 1–3, and 1–4.

The studies noted in these three tables indicate that a number of different types of mental disorders are found with sufficient frequency to warrant careful efforts to determine differential diagnoses in all women who seek treatment for LLPDD. These include major mood disorders, dysthymia, anxiety disorders, somatoform disorders, bulimia, substance use disorders, and personality disorders. Clinicians should also be alert to the possibility that other, nonmental medical disorders may be present. Frequently mentioned examples include seizure and thyroid disorders, cancer, lupus, anemia, and various infections.

For the most part, studies that report the rates of disorders occurring with LLPDD have not addressed the problem of differentiation of LLPDD as an additional diagnosis superimposed on an ongoing condition versus exacerbation of the ongoing condition. Neither have they taken into account the fact that other conditions may worsen during the late luteal phase of the menstrual cycle because of changes in the metabolism of medications during this time. When prospective daily ratings are considered over the entire menstrual cycle and clinical evaluations are conducted at two points in the cycle, the findings help clarify when there is *no* evidence of either an exacerbation of ongoing problems or the addition of new mood, behavioral, or physical problems. Often, however, a woman with a concurrent ongoing condition experiences some worsening of its symptoms or the appearance of new problems during the late luteal phase of the menstrual cycle. In such instances, it is often not possible to determine whether she would meet all of the criteria for LLPDD if the other medical condition were not present. Because no systematic studies were found that have focused on this issue, the frequency with which women would be found to have superimposed LLPDD is unclear.

Studies that have focused on lifetime comorbidity of mental disorders in women with LLPDD and no other current medical disorders usually indicate that these women have a higher rate of past mood and anxiety disorders than do women without severe premenstrual problems. Unfortunately, most of the studies that

Table 1–2. Evidence of current mental or other medical disorders in women with self-identified premenstrual problems

Reference	N subjects	Comments	Findings based on data from follicular phase
McMillan and Pihl 1987	28	Met criteria for premenstrual from major depressive syndrome	10 (37%) were found to have intermittent depression throughout the menstrual cycle.
Stout and Steege 1985	100	Sought evaluation for premenstrual syndrome (PMS) after passing telephone screening	64% showed evidence of problems during the follicular phase according to the Minnesota Multiphasic Personality Inventory (31% neurotic, 11% characterologic, 5% psychotic, 17% unclassified); 25% had clinically significant depression during the follicular phase according to the Beck Depression Inventory.
Hart and Russell 1986	31 12	Reported PMS Reported no problems	There were significant follicular phase differences in depression, anxiety, tension, and irritability, indicating that many of the women with PMS had problems throughout the cycle. No breakdown of numbers of women who accounted for the higher scores was provided.
Keye et al. 1986	68 34	Responded to a newspaper article about premenstrual problems. No complaints	Many medical conditions identified: hypertension (2), systemic lupus erythematosus (1), galactorrhea (5), breast mass (1), endometriosis (2), meningioma (1). 50% were currently under the care of a psychologist, but the number with current mental disorders was not noted.

(continued)

Table 1–2. Evidence of current mental or other medical disorders in women with self-identified premenstrual problems *(continued)*

Reference	*N* subjects	Comments	Findings based on data from follicular phase
Harrison et al. 1989b	195	Sought treatment for premenstrual anxiety, depression, or irritability and had completed at least one cycle of daily ratings and passed an initial telephone interview	87 (45%) had a current mental disorder.
Reid et al., unpublished data[a]	122	Referred to tertiary-care PMS clinic	30 women who had high follicular as well as luteal phase problems (12 had premenstrual exacerbation, 11 were high without exacerbation, 7 had drop in symptoms in late follicular phase only).
Severino et al. 1989	58	Self-referred for premenstrual difficulties	12 (21%) had a current anxiety or depressive disorder, 1 had another psychiatric disorder.

[a]Reid RL, Hahn PM, VanVugt DA: Characteristics of the menstrual cycle in women attending a premenstrual clinic, I: implications for diagnosis. Unpublished data, 1993.

Table 1–3. Evidence of premenstrual exacerbation of other mental disorders

Reference	Condition	Sample	Measures	Findings
Gladis and Walsh 1987	Bulimia	15 women who did not respond to placebo	Eating diaries	The mean scores for binges per day were compared for 5-day cycle segments; the segment just before menses was significantly higher than all other segments except the one just preceding it (days −10 to −5).
Bäckström et al. 1984	Epilepsy	Unknown	Seizure records	Cases were used to demonstrate that some women show a pattern of increased seizure frequency during the luteal phase, but the frequency with which this occurs was not noted.
Price et al. 1987	Bulimia	10 women with normal menstrual cycles	Weekly record of no. of binges for 2 months	All 10 increased binge eating; 5 showed marked increases (2 moderate and 3 small). The phase effect was significant for the total group.
Breier et al. 1986	Agoraphobia and panic attacks	43 with agoraphobia and panic attacks	Reports	51% of the women with agoraphobia had premenstrual exacerbation of symptoms.
Endicott and Halbreich 1988	Major depression	24 at depression clinic	Premenstrual Assessment Form[a]	83% reported worsening of depression and/or addition of symptoms premenstrually.
Slen 1984	Alcoholism	33 with regular cycles	Time of hospital admission	Significantly more subjects were admitted when they were menstruating, perhaps due to less control premenstrually.
Friedman et al. 1982	Mixed diagnosis	45 inpatients	Interview	28 (62%) met criteria for a premenstrual syndrome that differed from their usual symptoms.

[a]Halbreich et al. 1982.

Table 1–4. Evidence of premenstrual relapse or recurrence of mental disorder or other conditions

Reference	Condition	Sample	Measures	Findings
Brockington et al. 1988	Puerperal psychosis	8 patients	Relapse	10–17 relapses occurred during days –1 to –4 before menses.
Abramowitz et al. 1982	Depressive and schizophrenic disorders	39 depressed, 76 schizophrenic	Hospital admission	41% of the depressed women, but no schizophrenic women, had increased likelihood of having been admitted the day before or the day after menses started.
Hatotani et al. 1979	Periodic psychoses	47 with more than three episodes	Onsets	23 women had onsets regularly during the middle or later half of the menstrual cycle, none during the follicular period after menses, 3 during menses; 21 were irregular.
d'Orban and Dalton 1980	Violent criminal acts	50 with regular cycles	Criminal behavior	44% committed their offenses during the paramenstruum. Timing of offenses was unrelated to symptoms of premenstrual tension.
Luggin et al. 1984	Various conditions	121 acute admissions	Admission date	More admissions than expected took place during the menstrual period and fewer intermenstrually.

have reported on lifetime comorbid conditions have failed to clearly differentiate women with LLPDD only from those with exacerbations of ongoing mental disorders or concurrent comorbid mental disorders. As indicated in Table 1–5, few articles were found that made this distinction. The studies noted in Table 1–5 indicate that the incidence of comorbidity of prior disorders is relatively high, particularly with the major mood disorders.

There are many anecdotal reports that women who have severe mood problems that are limited to the late luteal phase are at risk for the development of other disorders, particularly depression. In the absence of prospective studies of women who meet the criteria for LLPDD without a concurrent Axis I or Axis II disorder, however, the degree of risk cannot be estimated.

Table 1–5. Evidence of prior lifetime comorbidity of other mental disorders with late luteal phase dysphoric disorder (LLPDD)

Reference	Subjects	Lifetime diagnosis
Harrison et al. 1989b	86 women who met criteria for LLPDD with no other Axis I or II disorders	70% prior major depressive disorder of 4 weeks or more 16% prior panic disorder 7% prior alcohol abuse 7% prior drug abuse
	61 control subjects with no premenstrual problems	41% prior major depressive disorder of 4 weeks or more 5% prior panic disorder 8% prior alcohol abuse 3% prior drug abuse
Pearlstein et al. 1990	78 women with no current Axis I or II disorders	46% prior major depressive disorder 69% prior major or minor depressive disorder 14% prior anxiety disorder
Ling and Brown 1990	83 women	48% history of depression
Severino et al. 1989	58 women	40% prior episode of anxiety or depressive disorder 4% prior substance abuse

Conclusions From the Literature Review

Clinicians and investigators have demonstrated that it is possible to identify women who meet the criteria for LLPDD in the absence of other current medical disorders. The differential diagnosis of LLPDD superimposed on another ongoing disorder, however, has been less well studied. The criteria proposed in DSM-III-R do not offer sufficient guidelines for determining whether clinical worsening during the late luteal phase reflects an exacerbation of another condition or superimposed LLPDD.

The studies reviewed here indicate that many women who seek treatment for premenstrual problems will not be found to have a clear-cut and distinct condition that meets the proposed criteria for LLPDD because the symptoms are not present, are not severe enough, or cannot be differentiated from some other chronic medical condition. If cycle changes in the specified clinical features are documented, the differential diagnosis of LLPDD from premenstrual changes or syndromes, as proposed in DSM-III-R, is primarily dependent on evidence of associated severe interference with social and occupational functioning. As is the case with other disorders in DSM-III-R, better guidelines for determining the necessary degree of "interference" or impairment are needed for this distinction to be made more reliably. If cyclic changes in clinical features are documented in an individual with another ongoing disorder, the diagnosis of superimposed LLPDD is more difficult to make, because the rules for attribution of impairment to the cyclic features (rather than the ongoing disorder) are not given in the proposed criteria.

For the most part, clinicians who have applied the proposed criteria for LLPDD have not expressed criticism over problems of judging how much change is clinically significant. This issue has been primarily one of great interest for research investigators, who wish to have more explicit guidelines to be assured that selected samples are similar.

The literature reports of comorbidity with other mental disorders, both current and lifetime, are numerous but need reevaluation in light of the methodological issues discussed in Chapter 2.

Some investigators have proposed that premenstrual dysphoric mood changes should simply be considered prodromal or residual manifestations of major mood disorders. Such a proposal is likely to obscure differences among groups of women with lifetime major mood disorders, some of whom also meet the criteria for LLPDD and some of whom do not. Certainly it would be premature to assume that every woman who meets the criteria for LLPDD will eventually have a major mood disorder. That two conditions are highly comorbid does not necessarily indicate that they are manifestations of the same condition. The levels of comorbidity reported here are not dissimilar to those reported for panic disorder or alcohol abuse and major mood disorders in women.

Practical Implications for Differential Diagnosis

What are the practical implications of the findings from the literature review for the practicing clinician or investigator selecting subjects for a particular study? First and foremost, there should be an awareness that most of the women who are referred or who present with self-defined premenstrual symptoms will not be found to meet the DSM-III-R criteria for LLPDD. This awareness should enable investigators to focus their diagnostic efforts on identifying other ongoing or episodic conditions that might account for the presenting complaints. The percentage of women who are found to meet the criteria for LLPDD will vary greatly, depending on the clinical setting (e.g., mental health, obstetric-gynecologic, or freestanding health care setting), referral sources, chief complaints, and diagnostic methodology.

A thorough general medical evaluation, including an assessment of possible current and lifetime mental disorders, is needed, and daily ratings recorded over several menstrual cycles are essential. It is also very helpful to examine each woman during both the follicular and the late luteal phases of the menstrual cycle, to contrast the clinical features that are present during the two phases. Because the week following menses is generally the time during which women have the fewest mood and behavior problems, the presence of problems during that week, coupled with daily ratings indicating ongoing problems, should alert clinicians to the need for more careful efforts to determine differential diagnoses. Women with LLPDD only should be essentially free of symptoms and impairment during that week. Women with superimposed LLPDD should no longer manifest most of the clinical features that characterized their premenstrual changes, although the features of an ongoing condition or disorder may be present. Information from significant others regarding the contrast between the premenstrual and postmenstrual phases of the cycle is also helpful in making the differential diagnosis.

Anecdotal reports suggest that initial efforts to treat LLPDD should focus on any ongoing conditions that have been identified, although no controlled studies have been performed in this manner. Such treatment may aid in the differential diagnosis of superimposed LLPDD versus an exacerbation of an ongoing condition. Even if the pattern after treatment indicates a continuation of premenstrual dysphoric changes, these may not be as troublesome once the ongoing condition is treated.

Some women will be found to have premenstrual dysphoric changes that are not severe enough to meet the impairment criteria for LLPDD, even though they may meet the symptom syndrome criteria. These women may not have the disorder, may be having a few atypical cycles that are less severe, or may have responded to the nonspecific therapeutic benefits of having professional attention focused on their concerns. In determining differential diagnoses in these women, it is often helpful for them to continue to monitor their condition over several additional cycles through the use of daily ratings.

Practical Implications for Monitoring the Condition

Given the high degree of lifetime comorbidity with other mental disorders, the clinician should continue to be alert to their possible occurrence, even after having made the diagnosis of uncomplicated LLPDD. Women who report that the severity and duration of premenstrual depression has increased noticeably over the past few cycles may be at risk for experiencing a prolonged period of major mood disorder. Women who have experiences of panic or isolated panic attacks that are limited to the premenstrual period and are increasing in severity or frequency over a period of several cycles may be at risk for the development of panic disorder. Clinicians should be especially alert for the possible development of substance use disorders in women who have a history of such disorders in themselves or in first-degree relatives. Periodic diagnostic reevaluation is needed to monitor the ongoing condition.

Conclusions

Some women have clinically significant problems with mood, behavior, and impairment in functioning that meet the proband DSM-III-R criteria for LLPDD. Identification of the disorder, however, requires careful differential diagnosis and ongoing monitoring of the condition. Most women who are evaluated in a clinical setting will be found to have some condition other than LLPDD.

References

Abramowitz ES, Baker AH, Fleiscler SF: Onset of depressive psychiatric crisis and the menstrual cycle. Am J Psychiatry 139:475–478, 1982

American Psychiatric Association: Diagnostic and Statistical Manual of Mental Disorders, 3rd Edition, Revised. Washington, DC, American Psychiatric Association, 1987

Bäckström T, Landgren S, Zetterland B, et al: Effects of ovarian steroid hormones on brain excitability and their relation to epilepsy seizure variation during the menstrual cycle, in Advances in Epileptology, Vol 15. Edited by Porter RJ, Mattson RH, Ward AA Jr, et al. New York, Raven Press, 1984, pp 269–277

Breier A, Charney DS, Heniger GR: Agoraphobia with panic attacks. Arch Gen Psychiatry 43:1029–1036, 1986

Brockington IF, Kelly A, Hall P, et al: Premenstrual relapse of puerperal psychosis. J Affect Disord 14:287–292, 1988

d'Orban PT, Dalton J: Violent crime and the menstrual cycle. Psychol Med 10:353–359, 1980

Endicott J, Halbreich U: Clinical significance of premenstrual dysphoric changes. J Clin Psychiatry 49:486–489, 1988

Friedman RC, Hurt SW, Charkin J, et al: Sexual histories and premenstrual affective syndrome in psychiatric inpatients. Am J Psychiatry 139:1484–1486, 1982

Gladis MM, Walsh BT: Premenstrual exacerbation of binge eating in bulimia. Psychiatry 144:1592–1595, 1987

Halbreich U, Endicott J, Schacht S, et al: The diversity of premenstrual changes as reflected in the Premenstrual Assessment Form (PAF). Acta Psychiatr Scand 65:46–65, 1982

Harrison WM, Endicott J, Nee J: Treatment of premenstrual depression with nortriptyline: a pilot study. J Clin Psychiatry 50:136–139, 1989a

Harrison WM, Endicott J, Nee J, et al: Characteristics of women seeking treatment for premenstrual syndrome. Psychosomatics 30:405–411, 1989b

Harrison WM, Sandberg D, Gorman J, et al: Provocation of panic with CO_2 inhalation in patients with premenstrual dysphoria. J Psychiatr Res 27:183–192, 1989c

Harrison WM, Endicott J, Nee J: Treatment of premenstrual dysphoria with alprazolam: a pilot study. Arch Gen Psychiatry 47:270–276, 1990

Hart WG, Russell JW: A prospective comparison study of premenstrual syndrome. Med J Aust 68:634–637, 1986

Hartmann L: Presidential address: reflections on human values and biopsychosocial integrations. Am J Psychiatry 149:1135–1141, 1992

Hatotani N, Nishikubo M, Iitayama I: Periodic psychosis in the female and the reproductive process, in Psychoneuroendocrinology in Reproduction. Edited by Zichella L, Pancheri P. New York, Elsevier North-Holland, 1979, pp 55–68

Hurt SW, Schnurr PP, Severino SK, et al: Late luteal phase dysphoric disorder in 670 women evaluated for premenstrual complaints. Am J Psychiatry 149:525–530, 1992

Keye WR Jr, Hammend DC, Strong T: Medical and psychological characteristics of women presenting with premenstrual problems. Obstet Gynecol 68:634–637, 1986

Ling FW, Brown CS: Clinical phenomenology of PMS: implications for the physician in a nonpsychiatric specialty area (abstract book #40). Paper presented at the Fourth National Institute of Mental Health International Research Conference on the Classification and Treatment of Mental Disorders in General Medical Settings, Bethesda, MD, June 1990

Luggin R, Bernsted L, Peterson B, et al: Acute psychiatric admission related to the menstrual cycle. Acta Psychiatr Scand 69:461–465, 1984

Magos AL, Brincat M, Studd JWW: Trend analysis. Am J Obstet Gynecol 155:277–282, 1986

McMillan MJ, Pihl RO: Premenstrual depression: a distinct entity. J Abnorm Psychol 92:149–154, 1987

Parry BL, Berga SL, Mostofi N, et al: Morning versus evening bright light treatment of late luteal phase dysphoric disorder. Am J Psychiatry 146:1215–1217, 1989

Pearlstein TH, Frank E, Rivera-Tovar A, et al: Prevalence of Axis I and Axis II disorders in women with late luteal phase dysphoric disorder. J Affect Disord 20:129–134, 1990

Price MA, Torem MS, DiMarzio LR: Premenstrual exacerbation of bulimia. Psychosomatics 28:378–379, 1987

Rausch JL, Janowsky DS, Golshan S, et al: Atenolol treatment of late luteal phase dysphoric disorder. J Affect Disord 15:141–147, 1988

Schnurr PP: Measuring amount of symptom change in the diagnosis of premenstrual syndrome. Psychological Assessment: J Consult Clin Psychol 1:277–283, 1989

Severino SK, Hurt SW, Shindledecker RD: Late luteal phase dysphoric disorder: spectral analysis of cyclic symptoms. Am J Psychiatry 146:1155–1160, 1989

Slen WW: A note on menstruation and hospital admission date of intoxicated women. Biol Psychiatry 19:1133–1136, 1984

Stone AB, Pearlstein T, Brown W: Fluoxetine in late luteal phase dysphoric disorder. Psychopharmacol Bull 26:331–335, 1990

Stout AL, Steege JF: Psychological assessment of women seeking treatment for premenstrual assessment. J Psychosom Res 29:621–629, 1985

Watkins PC, Williamson DA, Falhowski C: Prospective assessment of late luteal phase dysphoric disorder. Journal of Psychopathology and Behavioral Assessment 11:249–259, 1989

ℬ 2 ℬ

Consequences of Methodological Decisions in the Diagnosis of Late Luteal Phase Dysphoric Disorder

Paula P. Schnurr, Ph.D.
Stephen W. Hurt, Ph.D.
and Anna L. Stout, Ph.D.

> What is easiest to measure tends to get measured and called real, or important; what is harder to measure, even if as important, or more important, gets dismissed from reality, and gets measured and valued far less.
>
> Hartmann 1992, p. 1139

Late luteal phase dysphoric disorder (LLPDD) is a premenstrual condition defined in DSM-III-R (American Psychiatric Association 1987) by severe mood and other symptoms that repeatedly occur only in the luteal phase of the menstrual cycle. LLPDD is distinguished from most definitions of premenstrual syndrome (PMS) in several respects: 1) it requires at least one mood symptom to be among the five necessary for diagnosis, 2) these symptoms must be severe enough to cause functional impairment, and 3) they must not be an exacerbation of another disorder.

LLPDD is also distinguished from other diagnoses in DSM-III-R by its requirement that symptom changes be documented by prospective daily records in two menstrual cycles. On the one hand, this requirement is a significant advance in the diagnosis of premenstrual complaints. Previous research has shown that retrospective reports of symptoms that occur or increase in severity during the luteal phase and symptoms that discontinue or decrease in severity during the follicular phase are frequently not confirmed by prospective reports, even among treatment-seeking women (DeJong et al. 1985; Gallant et al. 1992; Hammarbäck et al. 1989; Hurt et al. 1992; Metcalf et al. 1989; Schnurr 1988, 1989a). On the other hand, the requirement for prospective confirmation can pose significant difficulties for analyzing prospective records in order to make a diagnosis. DSM-III-R does not specify how to compute the change from the follicular to the luteal phase or how to determine when the amount of change is great enough to warrant a diagnosis.

Over the past decade, researchers have recommended a number of different methods that sometimes vary greatly in the extent to which they agree on the diagnosis of LLPDD (Gallant et al. 1992; Hurt et al. 1992) or PMS in general (Metcalf et al. 1989; Schnurr 1989a). By showing that decisions about what constitutes a case differ according to the method used, these findings beg the question of which method to use, that is, of which is the "best," or the most valid.

The obvious way to examine a question of diagnostic validity is to compare a diagnostic test or tests with a true (or accepted as true) indicator of the disorder in question. Unfortunately, there is no such "gold standard" for diagnoses related to the menstrual cycle. The next best strategy, as suggested by Feighner and colleagues (1972), is to establish validity in five phases: 1) clinical description, 2) laboratory studies, 3) delimitation from other disorders, 4) follow-up studies, and 5) family studies. Presumably, individuals who are validly diagnosed share not only a common set of symptoms that distinguish them from individuals with other disorders, but are also relatively homogeneous in terms of features such as demographic background, precipitating factors, biological and psychological test findings, course of symptoms, and family comorbidity.

To our knowledge, only one previous group of investigators has followed this logic in an investigation of methodological issues in the diagnosis of PMS. Hammarbäck and colleagues (1989) varied the number of days used to define follicular and luteal phases for comparison (from 5 to 10 days each) and found that decreasing the number of days resulted in poorer discrimination between diagnostic groups in terms of their lifetime history of psychiatric disorders and a measure of neuroticism.[1]

Applying the strategy of Feighner and colleagues (1972) to the problem of validating methods for the diagnosis of LLPDD would involve an examination of how varying the method used for analyzing change affects the homogeneity of groups defined as having and as not having the disorder. Here we report one such study, which was conducted with the data set compiled by the DSM-IV Work Group on LLPDD. In initial analyses of this data set, the prevalence of symptoms and overall diagnosis in treatment-seeking women were estimated as a function of four methods used to analyze change (Hurt et al. 1992). The prevalence of LLPDD ranged from 14% for the absolute severity method (Eckerd et al. 1989) to 45% for trend analysis (Magos and Studd 1986), with the effect size method (Schnurr 1988) and a variant of the percent change method (Eckerd et al. 1989) falling in between.

In the study described here, we defined LLPDD according to several existing methods and examined symptom severity, demographic characteristics, and psychiatric history in the resulting "LLPDD" and "non-LLPDD" groups. The methods chosen to analyze change were absolute severity, effect size, and percent change,

---

[1] The use of longer-phase definitions unfortunately may make it difficult for a woman who has a short cycle to have a sufficient number of follicular days for analysis. Attempts to adhere to the definition in such cases may lead to the inclusion of menstrual days or periovulatory days. On balance, the use of 6- or 7-day phases may be optimal, even though it may increase diagnostic heterogeneity somewhat.

defined as a luteal phase increase of 30% of scale length (Rubinow and Roy-Byrne 1984).

It would be reasonable to expect that the most valid method would yield the greatest separation between groups in symptom severity. In particular, the DSM-III-R requirements for symptoms to cause serious functional interference and not to be an exacerbation of an ongoing disorder led us to expect that the most valid method would yield cases with the highest severity ratings in the luteal phase and the lowest severity ratings in the follicular phase. Given that the absolute severity method was the only one of the three methods that explicitly incorporated these requirements into its diagnostic criteria, we expected that it would produce the greatest differences between groups in follicular phase averages, luteal phase averages, and the difference between the two phases as represented by an effect size.

We turned to the PMS literature to make predictions about demographic and psychiatric variables, because little information exists about the correlates of prospectively defined LLPDD. Among women who seek treatment for PMS, those whose retrospective reports are confirmed by prospective diaries tend to be younger than those whose reports are not confirmed (DeJong et al. 1985; Schnurr 1988). Few other demographic correlates of prospectively defined PMS have been observed, although Sanders and colleagues (1983) found that women with retrospectively defined PMS, 73% of whom met prospective criteria, had an increased likelihood of being married, having children, and being unemployed. Freeman and colleagues (1988) have also found the severity of prospectively defined PMS to be negatively associated with age and positively associated with number of children.

There are a number of studies on the relationship between PMS and psychiatric disorders. Data on this subject are especially relevant to a study of methods for diagnosing LLPDD, because DSM-III-R specifies that LLPDD must not be an exacerbation of the symptoms of another disorder. As indicated in Chapter 1, earlier reports in the literature relying on retrospective reports for the diagnosis of premenstrual symptoms indicated a strong relationship with psychiatric disorders. For example, Stout and colleagues

(1986) examined lifetime diagnoses in treatment-seeking women who retrospectively reported premenstrual difficulties. These women were more likely than women in a matched community sample to meet DSM-III (American Psychiatric Association 1980) criteria for dysthymia, phobia, obsessive-compulsive disorder, and alcohol or drug abuse or dependence.

If we confine ourselves to studies in which treatment-seeking women who meet prospective criteria for PMS were compared with those who do not (in order to mimic the clinical necessity of differential diagnosis), we find that women with PMS have a decreased likelihood of lifetime psychiatric disorders. West (1989) found that women with PMS who had the greatest amount of remission from the luteal to the follicular phase were the least likely to have a history of treatment for psychiatric disorders. DeJong and colleagues (1985) found a significantly lower prevalence of lifetime psychiatric diagnoses in women whose retrospective reports were prospectively confirmed (45%) than in women whose reports were not confirmed (88%). Hammarbäck and colleagues (1989) also found a lower percentage of lifetime psychiatric disorders in women whose prospective charting reflected symptoms that were restricted to the premenstruum than in women who had premenstrual worsening of chronic symptoms or whose symptoms had no correlation with the menstrual cycle. Thus, we might expect that the most valid method for diagnosing LLPDD would be one that identifies women who have a decreased history of lifetime psychiatric disorders relative to women who do not meet prospective diagnostic criteria for LLPDD. The absolute severity method would seem best suited for this purpose because it requires a predominantly asymptomatic follicular phase, which is unlikely in a woman with a chronic psychiatric disorder, especially if the disorder is current.

Data on the relationship between PMS and affective disorders are also relevant because of the diagnostic requirement for women with LLPDD to have at least one mood symptom. There is little known about major affective disorder in treatment-seeking women who meet the prospective diagnostic criteria for LLPDD relative to those who do not. In DeJong and colleagues' (1985) sample, major affective disorder was present in two-thirds of those who had a psychiatric disorder in both the confirmed PMS group and in the unconfirmed PMS group. Given the markedly decreased likelihood of any psychiatric disorder in the study by DeJong et al., however, PMS was associated with a decreased likelihood of lifetime major affective disorders relative to other disorders only (odds ratio = 0.12; 95% confidence interval = 0.03–0.52) or other disorders or no disorder (odds ratio = 0.31; 95% confidence interval = 0.10–0.93). (Note that these estimates are based on our own analyses of the data of DeJong et al.) This suggests that the most valid method for diagnosing LLPDD would be associated with the lowest prevalence of affective disorder.

Our previous study (Hurt et al. 1992) only partially addressed questions of the relationship between LLPDD and psychiatric disorders. A history of psychiatric disorders only was associated with an increased risk of LLPDD, as defined according to all methods except the absolute severity method, for which the risk was nonsignificantly decreased (relative risk = 0.80; 95% confidence interval = 0.52–1.22). The presence of a current psychiatric disorder was not associated with an increased or a decreased risk of LLPDD according to any method. We did not find an association between major affective disorder and LLPDD, except for an increased risk of LLPDD diagnosed by trend analysis in women with past disorders only. In this chapter, we expand on these analyses by examining lifetime history of psychiatric disorder, as well as other types of disorders, in greater detail.

Because diagnoses made according to each method overlap, we also created aggregate diagnostic groups in a manner similar to that used by Hammarbäck and colleagues (1989) to distinguish "pure" from "aggravated" PMS. First, we determined whether a woman experienced change according to scoring criteria for either the effect size or the percent change method. If a woman did not meet either criterion for change, she was considered to have no change. Next, we divided the number of women with change, on the basis of whether they met the scoring criteria of the absolute severity method, into the number of women with absolute severity and change and change-only groups (LLPDD-ASC and LLPDD-

CO, respectively). Women with change only could be expected to be more likely to have exacerbation of ongoing symptoms in the luteal phase, or instead, to have only mild symptoms in the luteal phase. In either case, we expected that the LLPDD-CO group would fall in between the LLPDD-ASC and no-change groups in terms of psychiatric history and demographic variables.

Methods

A full description of our methods can be found in the study by Hurt and colleagues (1992). Following is a brief description and information about several differences between this and our initial report.

Subjects

Subjects were drawn from one of five PMS clinics located in the north and southeastern United States. All subjects kept daily prospective ratings of LLPDD symptoms for at least two menstrual cycles and had cycles between 22 and 35 days in length (mean = 26.9; standard deviation [SD] = 4.0). They were selected from the 670 subjects in our initial report if they had data on two menstrual cycles only ($n = 628$) or if they had data on more than two cycles but a diagnosis based on their first two cycles was consistent with the diagnosis they would have received by considering all of the cycles available ($n = 20$).

The 648 subjects did not differ significantly from those in our initial report (Hurt et al. 1992). On average, they were 33.8 years old (SD = 5.6) and had 1.3 children (SD = 1.2) and 1.9 pregnancies (SD = 1.6). Almost 70% were employed, 95.5% were white, and 43.9% had graduated from college.

Procedures

Diagnoses were based on the analysis of prospective daily ratings for the 10 DSM-III-R symptom criteria for LLPDD. Ratings were typically made on a 6-point scale on which 1 indicated minimal or no symptoms and 6 indicated maximum intensity of symptoms. Diagnoses were made according to three methods, each of which compared ratings on menstrual cycle follicular days 5–10 with ratings during the last 6 luteal days of the menstrual cycle in two consecutive menstrual cycles. For each method, a woman received a diagnosis if she had five or more symptoms that met the criteria for that method; at least one of these symptoms had to be marked affective lability, anger/irritability, anxiety/tension, or depression.

For the absolute severity method, the criteria required that no more than 2 days were rated above 2 in the follicular phase and at least 1 day was rated above 4 in the luteal phase. For the effect size method, the difference between the luteal phase average and the follicular phase average, divided by the cycle SD, had to be ≥ 1.0. For the percent change method, the difference between the luteal phase average and the follicular phase average had to be ≥ 30% of the scale length; note that this differs from the 75% of baseline used in our initial study but is consistent with most uses of this method (e.g., DeJong et al. 1985).

Psychiatric history data were derived from structured or clinical interviews as described by Hurt and colleagues (1992). In addition to the occurrence of any disorder, we examined three subcategories: mood disorders (any DSM-III-R mood disorder, including major depression, dysthymia, and bipolar disorder), anxiety disorders (including generalized anxiety disorder, panic disorder, and phobias), and other Axis I and Axis II disorders. We report the data separately for current disorder (including past), past only, and lifetime.

Data Analysis

Differences between diagnostic groups in symptom severity levels were tested by *t* tests for comparisons involving women with LLPDD (cases) and women without LLPDD (non-cases) according to each of the three methods. One-way analysis of variance (ANOVA) was used to compare differences in symptom scores between the aggregate diagnostic groups, and Tukey tests (Kirk

1982) were used to compare means. In both instances, the difference between LLPDD and non-LLPDD groups was computed as the effect size, d, the proportion of a standard deviation by which groups differed. The non-LLPDD or no-change group was used as the reference group (depending on the analysis), so that a positive effect size indicates that cases had a higher score.

Differences between diagnostic groups in categorically scaled demographic variables and all psychiatric variables were computed as odds ratios, using "non-LLPDD" or "no change" as the reference category, depending on the analysis. For continuously scaled demographic variables, we used the effect size index, d, computed as described above.

Results

Differences Among Scoring Methods

The prevalence of LLPDD according to each method is shown in Table 2–1. The effect size method yielded the greatest number of cases (36.6%), and the absolute severity method yielded the least (13.3%). The percent change method yielded an intermediate number (21.9%). Table 2–1 also shows the percentage of cases that met LLPDD criteria for one of the two cycles. These data show that a number of subjects who were diagnosed as not having LLPDD actually had notable symptomatology at least some of the time. Still, almost two-thirds of treatment-seeking women did not meet the criteria of the absolute severity method

Table 2–1. Occurrence of diagnosis of late luteal phase dysphoric disorder by scoring method

Cycle	Absolute severity		Effect size		Percent change	
	%	n	%	n	%	n
Both	13.3	86	36.6	237	21.9	142
One only	24.2	157	34.4	223	29.2	189
Neither	62.5	405	29.0	188	48.9	317

for even one cycle, although the percentage that failed to meet the other criteria for even one cycle was much lower—29.0% for the effect size method and 48.9% for the percent change method.

Table 2–2 shows information about symptom severity in cases and non-cases defined according to each method. Regardless of the method used, cases differed markedly from non-cases in average luteal and follicular phase symptom scores. Cases also differed from non-cases in the amount of symptom worsening, computed as the effect size of the difference between the luteal phase average and the follicular phase average. Differences between cases and non-cases according to each method appeared to be similar across cycles for all measures.

It is not possible to compare scoring methods statistically because of the partial overlap between diagnostic groups according to each method. Visual inspection of the means and between-group effect sizes, however, suggests several interesting patterns. The best separation between groups in luteal phase symptomatology was for the absolute severity method; the poorest was for the effect size method. Contrary to our expectation, the absolute severity method produced the poorest separation between cases and non-cases in follicular phase symptomatology, and the effect size method produced the best. In addition, the average follicular phase score in cases was lower according to the effect size and the percent change methods. The amount of symptom worsening was greatest for the effect size and the percent change scoring methods.

Tables 2–3 and 2–4 show the results of analyses of the demographic and psychiatric data. In terms of the demographic data in Table 2–3, the only statistically significant difference between cases and non-cases was in age, and only for diagnoses made according to the absolute severity and the percent change methods. As expected, younger women were more likely than older women to be diagnosed with LLPDD. For each method, cases were approximately one-fourth of an SD younger than non-cases.

The psychiatric history data in Table 2–4 show few differences between cases and non-cases as defined by any scoring method.

Table 2–2. Symptom measures by phase as a function of scoring method and diagnosis of late luteal phase dysphoric disorder

Phase	Absolute severity			Effect size			Percent change		
	Yes	No[a]	d	Yes	No[a]	d	Yes	No[a]	d
Luteal mean									
Cycle 1	3.89 (0.76)	2.63 (0.92)	1.26	3.35 (0.88)	2.48 (0.92)	0.87	3.78 (0.73)	2.52 (0.88)	1.26
Cycle 2	3.90 (0.84)	2.48 (0.88)	1.43	3.20 (0.89)	2.36 (0.92)	0.85	3.61 (0.79)	2.41 (0.88)	1.21
Follicular mean									
Cycle 1	1.43 (0.41)	1.59 (0.68)	−0.25*	1.34 (0.40)	1.70 (0.73)	−0.55	1.36 (0.41)	1.63 (0.69)	−0.42
Cycle 2	1.43 (0.42)	1.63 (0.68)	−0.30**	1.39 (0.42)	1.73 (0.74)	−0.52	1.38 (0.38)	1.67 (0.71)	−0.44
Effect size									
Cycle 1	1.60 (0.44)	0.91 (0.64)	1.05	1.54 (0.38)	0.69 (0.58)	1.29	1.68 (0.36)	0.81 (0.59)	1.32
Cycle 2	1.58 (0.39)	0.76 (0.61)	1.26	1.41 (0.37)	0.55 (0.56)	1.32	1.56 (0.31)	0.67 (0.58)	1.37

Note. Standard deviations appear in parentheses. The statistic *d* indicates the effect size of the difference between late luteal phase dysphoric disorder (LLPDD) and non-LLPDD groups (see text).

[a] Reference category. *$P < .05$; **$P < .01$ for two-tailed *t* test (df = 646). All other differences are $P < .001$.

Table 2–3. Demographic correlates of late luteal phase dysphoric disorder by scoring method

Characteristic	Absolute severity			Effect size			Percent change		
	Yes	No[a]	d	Yes	No[a]	d	Yes	No[a]	d
Age (years)	32.54 (4.91)	33.94 (5.66)	−0.25*	33.48 (5.19)	33.91 (5.82)	−0.08	32.71 (4.99)	34.04 (5.73)	−0.24*
N children	1.23 (1.24)	1.32 (1.24)	−0.07	1.26 (1.23)	1.32 (1.20)	−0.06	1.26 (1.24)	1.31 (1.20)	−0.05
N pregnancies	1.71 (1.47)	1.90 (1.62)	−0.12	1.81 (1.60)	1.92 (1.20)	−0.07	1.89 (1.68)	1.87 (1.58)	0.01

Characteristic	Absolute severity				Effect size				Percent change			
	Yes	No	OR	95% CI	Yes	No	OR	95% CI	Yes	No	OR	95% CI
Employed	67.4	69.4	0.91	0.56, 1.48	70.5	68.4	1.10	0.78, 1.56	68.3	69.4	0.95	0.64, 1.42
Minority race	4.7	4.4	1.04	0.36, 3.09	4.6	4.4	1.06	0.49, 2.29	5.6	4.2	1.38	0.60, 3.18
College graduate	40.7	47.0	0.77	0.49, 1.23	45.1	46.7	0.94	0.68, 1.29	41.5	47.4	0.79	0.54, 1.15

Note. Means (SDs) are presented for age, number of children, and number of pregnancies. Percentages (% yes) are presented for work status, race, and education. OR = odds ratio; CI = confidence interval.
[a] Reference category.
* $P < .05$.

Table 2–4. Psychiatric correlates of late luteal phase dysphoric disorder by scoring method

Type of disorder	Absolute severity				Effect size				Percent change			
	Yes	No[a]	OR	95% CI	Yes	No[a]	OR	95% CI	Yes	No[a]	OR	95% CI
Lifetime diagnosis												
Mood disorder	53.5	51.8	1.07	0.68, 1.69	56.5	49.4	1.33	0.97, 1.84	57.0	50.6	1.30	0.89, 1.89
Anxiety disorder	17.4	24.9	0.64	0.35, 1.15	24.5	23.6	1.05	0.72, 1.52	19.0	25.3	0.69	0.43, 1.10
Other Axis I or II	17.4	23.1	0.70	0.39, 1.27	21.1	23.3	0.89	0.60, 1.31	19.0	23.3	0.77	0.49, 1.23
Any disorder	61.6	67.8	0.76	0.48, 1.22	69.6	65.5	1.21	0.86, 1.71	70.4	66.0	1.23	0.82, 1.84
Current diagnosis												
Mood disorder	15.1	13.0	1.19	0.63, 2.26	11.4	14.4	0.77	0.47, 1.25	14.1	13.0	1.09	0.64, 1.87
Anxiety disorder	8.1	13.5	0.57	0.25, 1.27	11.4	13.6	0.82	0.50, 1.33	9.2	13.8	0.63	0.34, 1.17
Other Axis I or II	7.0	9.6	0.71	0.29, 1.69	6.3	10.9	0.55	0.30, 1.01	7.0	9.9	0.69	0.34, 1.40
Any disorder	26.7	27.8	0.95	0.57, 1.59	24.5	29.4	0.78	0.54, 1.12	27.5	27.7	0.99	0.65, 1.50
Past-only diagnosis												
Mood disorder	38.4	38.8	0.98	0.62, 1.57	45.1	35.0	1.52*	1.10, 2.12	43.0	37.5	1.25	0.86, 1.83
Anxiety disorder	9.3	11.4	0.80	0.37, 1.73	13.1	10.0	1.36	0.83, 2.23	9.9	11.5	0.84	0.46, 1.56
Other Axis I or II	10.5	13.5	0.75	0.36, 1.55	14.8	12.2	1.25	0.79, 1.99	12.0	13.4	0.88	0.50, 1.55
Any disorder	34.9	40.0	0.80	0.50, 1.29	45.1	36.0	1.46*	1.06, 2.03	43.0	38.3	1.21	0.83, 1.77

Note. OR = odds ratio; CI = confidence interval.
[a]Reference category.
*$P < .05$.

LLPDD as defined by the absolute severity method decreased the likelihood of lifetime psychiatric disorders by 24%. In contrast, LLPDD as defined by either the effect size or the percent change method increased the likelihood of lifetime psychiatric disorders by more than 20%. None of the odds ratios differed from 1.0, however, and their overlapping confidence intervals suggest that they do not differ from each other. The only differences between cases and non-cases in any of the psychiatric variables were for cases defined by the effect size method to have an approximately 50% increase in likelihood of any psychiatric disorder and mood disorder in the past only.

Agreement Among Scoring Methods

Information about agreement among scoring methods is shown in Table 2–5. Clearly, the differences in prevalence among methods are not merely the result of the absolute severity method being the most conservative and the effect size method being the most liberal. The methods also disagreed about what does and does not constitute a case. There was statistically significant agreement among all methods, but agreement was generally poor between the absolute severity and the effect size methods, both overall and in each cycle ($\kappa < 0.40$). Agreement between

Table 2–5. κ Coefficients for agreement among scoring methods

Cycle	Effect size	Percent change
Both		
Absolute severity	0.33	0.52
Effect size	—	0.64
Cycle 1		
Absolute severity	0.35	0.60
Effect size	—	0.62
Cycle 2		
Absolute severity	0.36	0.55
Effect size	—	0.66

Note. All κ values are statistically significant at $P < .001$.

the absolute severity and the percent change methods and between the effect size and the percent change methods was better, but still only moderate.

Table 2–6 shows how information provided by the three scoring methods was used to create aggregate diagnostic groups. Just over one-third of the women ($n = 239$; 36.9%) were classified as having LLPDD, most of them ($n = 164$) by change criteria only. It is remarkable, however, that over 60% of the sample did not meet criteria according to any method.

Differences Among Aggregate Diagnostic Groups

Table 2–7 shows the symptom severity measures of the three aggregate diagnostic groups. One-way ANOVAs showed that the groups differed significantly on all measures in both cycles: luteal means ($F[2,645] = 110.5$ and 114.8; $Ps < .001$, respectively), follicular means ($F[2,645] = 24.1$ and 21.5; $Ps < .001$, respectively), and follicular-luteal effect sizes ($F[2,645] = 210.1$ and 239.7; $Ps < .001$, respectively). Tukey tests at $P < .05$ showed that both LLPDD groups had higher luteal phase scores, lower follicular phase scores, and larger follicular-luteal phase effect sizes

Table 2–6. Definition of aggregate diagnostic groups

Scoring method					
Absolute severity	Effect size	Percent change	n	%	Aggregate diagnostic group
Yes	Yes	Yes	68	10.5	Absolute severity
Yes	Yes	No	7	1.1	and change
Yes	No	Yes	0	0.0	$n = 75$ (11.6%)
No	Yes	Yes	72	11.1	Change only
No	Yes	No	90	13.9	$n = 164$ (25.3%)
No	No	Yes	2	0.3	
Yes	No	No	11	1.7	No change
No	No	No	398	61.4	$n = 409$ (63.1%)

LLPDD $n = 239$ (36.9%)

than women without LLPDD. The LLPDD-CO group also had smaller effect sizes and lower luteal phase scores in both cycles than did the LLPDD-ASC group. The two LLPDD groups, however, were almost identical in follicular phase symptomatology. This suggests that women who meet change criteria without meeting the criteria of the absolute severity method have milder luteal phase symptoms and less severe, but demonstrable, LLPDD, rather than a premenstrual exacerbation of chronic symptoms. If present, such symptom elevations would have appeared during the follicular phase as well.

Table 2–8 shows that there were no differences between the aggregate groups in demographic characteristics. Table 2–9 shows that the LLPDD-CO group was less likely than the no-change group to have a current psychiatric disorder other than a mood or anxiety disorder and was more likely to have a history of any disorder, especially a mood disorder. Contrary to our expectations, the LLPDD-ASC group did not differ from the no-change group, even in likelihood of any current psychiatric disorder.

Table 2–7. Symptom severity measures by cycle as a function of aggregate diagnostic group

| | | LLPDD group | | | |
| | No change[a] | Absolute severity and change | | Change only | |
Cycle	Mean (SD)	Mean (SD)	d	Mean (SD)	d
Luteal mean					
Cycle 1	2.47_1 (0.91)	4.01_2 (0.72)	1.53	3.05_3 (0.79)	0.58
Cycle 2	2.36_1 (0.92)	3.94_2 (0.79)	1.60	2.87_3 (0.71)	0.52
Follicular mean					
Cycle 1	1.70_1 (0.72)	1.37_2 (0.37)	−0.51	1.34_2 (0.44)	−0.62
Cycle 2	1.73_1 (0.74)	1.38_2 (0.39)	−0.53	1.40_2 (0.44)	−0.50
Effect size					
Cycle 1	0.69_1 (0.58)	1.71_2 (0.35)	1.55	1.46_3 (0.37)	1.17
Cycle 2	0.55_1 (0.56)	1.65_2 (0.33)	1.69	1.29_3 (0.34)	1.14

Note. Row means that do not share a common subscript differ by at least $P < .05$.
LLPDD = late luteal phase dysphoric disorder.
[a]Reference category.

Additional Issues

The relative lack of differences we observed in demographic characteristics and psychiatric history between women with LLPDD and women without LLPDD led us to the additional analyses described here.

Consistency Over Cycles

As noted above, many women classified as non-cases according to a given method actually met DSM-III-R criteria according to that method for one of the two cycles studied. For the analyses involving all scoring methods, the prevalence of psychiatric disorders among these women typically fell in between the prevalence in the non-LLPDD and LLPDD groups. We excluded these partial cases from the non-LLPDD groups for each of the three scoring methods and reanalyzed the psychiatric data. Doing so

Table 2–8. Demographic correlates of late luteal phase dysphoric disorder (LLPDD) by aggregate diagnostic group

		LLPDD group					
	No change[a]	Absolute severity and change			Change only		
Characteristic	Mean (SD)	Mean (SD)	d		Mean (SD)	d	
Age (years)	33.93 (5.81)	32.61 (5.13)	−0.18		33.84 (5.23)	−0.02	
N children	1.33 (1.20)	1.18 (1.22)	−0.12		1.28 (1.24)	−0.04	
N pregnancies	1.92 (1.60)	1.60 (1.46)	−0.20		1.90 (1.65)	0.00	
	%	%	OR	95% CI	%	OR	95% CI
Employed	68.5	69.3	1.04	0.61, 1.78	70.7	1.11	0.75, 1.65
Minority race	4.4	4.0	0.91	0.26, 3.15	4.9	1.11	0.47, 2.61
College graduate	46.7	45.3	0.95	0.58, 1.55	45.1	0.94	0.65, 1.35

Note. Means (SDs) are presented for age, number of children, and number of pregnancies. Percentages (% yes) are presented for work status, race, and education. OR = odds ratio. CI = confidence interval.
[a]Reference category.

had little effect on the odds ratios associated with LLPDD defined by either the absolute severity or the percent change method. For the effect size analyses, however, excluding partial cases from the non-LLPDD group decreased the prevalence in this group of any past-only disorder (from 36.0% to 30.3%) and mood disorder, both past only (from 35.0% to 30.3%) and lifetime (from 49.4% to 45.2%). There also was an increased prevalence in the redefined non-LLPDD group of any current disorder (from 29.4% to 34.6%) and current disorder other than mood or anxiety (from 10.9% to 13.8%). These changes in

Table 2–9. Psychiatric correlates of late luteal phase dysphoric disorder (LLPDD) by aggregate diagnostic group

| | | LLPDD group | | | | | |
| | | Absolute severity and change | | | Change only | | |
Type of disorder	No change[a] %	%	OR	95% CI	%	OR	95% CI
Lifetime diagnosis							
Mood disorder	49.1	56.0	1.32	0.80, 2.16	57.3	1.39	0.96, 2.00
Anxiety disorder	23.7	17.3	0.67	0.36, 1.28	27.4	1.22	0.81, 1.84
Other Axis I or							
Axis II	23.2	18.7	0.76	0.40, 1.42	22.0	0.93	0.60, 1.43
Any disorder	65.3	64.0	0.95	0.57, 1.58	72.6	1.41	0.94, 2.10
Current diagnosis							
Mood disorder	14.2	14.7	1.04	0.52, 2.09	10.4	0.70	0.39, 1.24
Anxiety disorder	13.7	8.0	0.55	0.23, 1.32	12.8	0.93	0.54, 1.59
Other Axis I or							
Axis II	11.0	8.0	0.70	0.29, 1.71	5.5	0.47[*]	0.22, 0.98
Any disorder	29.3	26.7	0.88	0.50, 1.52	23.8	0.75	0.49, 1.14
Past-only diagnosis							
Mood disorder	35.0	41.3	1.31	0.80, 2.17	47.0	1.65[*]	1.14, 2.38
Anxiety disorder	10.0	9.3	0.92	0.40, 2.15	14.6	1.54	0.90, 2.64
Other Axis I or							
Axis II	12.2	10.7	0.86	0.39, 1.89	16.5	1.41	0.85, 2.35
Any disorder	35.9	37.3	1.06	0.64, 1.77	48.8	1.70[**]	1.18, 2.45

Note. OR = odds ratio. CI = confidence interval.
[a]Reference category.
[*]$P < .05$; [**]$P < .01$.

turn increased the odds associated with LLPDD diagnosed by the effect size method of lifetime mood disorder (odds ratio = 1.58; 95% confidence interval = 1.07, 2.32), any past-only disorder (odds ratio = 1.89; 95% confidence interval = 1.26, 2.83), and past-only mood disorder (odds ratio = 1.89; 95% confidence interval = 1.26, 2.83). The changes also decreased the odds associated with LLPDD of current disorder other than mood or anxiety (odds ratio = 0.42; 95% confidence interval = 0.22, 0.82) and any current disorder (odds ratio = 0.62; 95% confidence interval = 0.40, 0.93).

Homogeneity of Non-LLPDD Women

When reviewing the analyses involving aggregate diagnostic groups, we reconsidered the assignment of the 11 women who met the criteria of the absolute severity method but neither of the change criteria. They originally were classified as "no change" according to our analysis plan. We believed, however, that it would be useful to examine differences between them and the other women in the no-change group, even though the relatively low power of these comparisons would make it difficult to detect even moderate differences. These women were comparable to the no-change subgroup in follicular phase symptomatology, with nonsignificantly higher ratings in both cycles. They were more symptomatic during the luteal phase of both cycles (cycle 1: 3.12 versus 2.45, t [407] = 2.40, $P < .05$; cycle 2: 3.61 versus 2.32, t [407] = 4.72, $P < .001$). Overall, the effect size of the change between follicular and luteal phase ratings was higher in the absolute severity subgroup (cycle 1: 0.88 versus 0.69, t [12.74] < 2.20, $P < .05$; cycle 2: 1.10 versus 0.53, t [407] = 3.36, $P < .001$).

There was one difference between the two no-change subgroups on the demographic variables. The absolute severity subgroup was much less likely to have graduated from college (odds ratio = 0.11; 95% confidence interval = 0.01, 0.86). There were no significant differences in likelihood of psychiatric disorders. There was a nonsignificant trend for the absolute severity subgroup to be less likely to have any past-only disorder (18.2% versus 36.4%) or past-only mood disorder (18.2% versus 35.4%), yet the groups were comparable in likelihood of any current disorder and current mood disorder (27.3 versus 29.4 and 18.2 versus 14.1, respectively).

Effects of Follicular Phase Symptomatology on Likelihood of Current Psychiatric Disorder

We had expected that the requirement of the absolute severity method for a generally asymptomatic follicular phase would result in fewer women who met the criteria of that method to have a current psychiatric disorder. Our failure to find this difference caused us to wonder about the relationship between follicular phase symptomatology in general and likelihood of current psychiatric disorders. We addressed this question first by examining follicular phase symptoms averaged across both cycles in women with and without a current psychiatric disorder. We found that women who had a current psychiatric disorder reported higher follicular phase symptoms than women who did not have a current disorder (1.75 versus 1.52, t [646] = 4.34, P = .001). This also was true for specific diagnostic categories: mood (1.73 versus 1.57, t [646] = 2.47, P < .05) and other Axis I and II disorders (1.74 versus 1.57, t [646] = 2.15, P < .05).

Next, we divided the number of subjects with LLPDD according to each scoring method into two groups on the basis of follicular phase symptoms. A subject was designated "low" if she had a follicular phase average of 1.5 or less. Otherwise, she was designated "high." The number of women with LLPDD in each of our three groups who had low follicular phase symptoms was as follows: absolute severity method, n = 57, 66.3%; effect size method, n = 174, 73.4%; and percent change method, n = 100, 70.4%.

Table 2–10 shows that the likelihood of a current psychiatric disorder was significantly lower in women with low follicular phase symptoms than in those with higher symptoms. For the effect size and the percent change methods, women with low follicular phase symptoms also had a significantly decreased likelihood of current Axis I disorders other than mood or Axis II disorders.

Table 2–10. Current psychiatric disorder and follicular phase symptoms in women with late luteal phase dysphoric disorder

Type of disorder	Absolute severity				Effect size				Percent change			
	Low	High[a]	OR	95% CI	Low	High[a]	OR	95% CI	Low	High[a]	OR	95% CI
Mood disorder	12.3	20.7	0.54	0.16, 1.78	10.9	12.7	0.84	0.34, 2.03	11.0	21.4	0.45	0.17, 1.19
Anxiety disorder	5.3	13.8	0.35	0.07, 1.67	9.2	17.5	0.48	0.21, 1.10	8.0	11.9	0.64	0.20, 2.10
Other Axis I or II	3.5	13.8	0.23	0.04, 1.32	4.0	12.7	0.29*	0.10, 0.83	4.0	14.3	0.25*	0.07, 0.94
Any disorder	17.5	4.8	0.26**	0.10, 0.71	20.1	36.5	0.44**	0.23, 0.82	21.0	42.9	0.35**	0.16, 0.77

Note. "Low" and "high" refer to the percentage of women in each group who have a current disorder. Low = follicular phase average ≤1.5.
High = follicular phase symptom average > 1.5. OR = odds ratio. CI = confidence interval.
[a]Reference category.
*$P < .05$; **$P < .01$.

Discussion

The study described in this chapter was intended to provide information about the validity of three methods for scoring symptom changes in the diagnosis of LLPDD. Using a logic proposed by Feighner and colleagues (1972), we hypothesized that the most valid method would yield the best discrimination between women with and without LLPDD in symptom severity, demographic characteristics, and psychiatric history. We had expected that the absolute severity method (Eckerd et al. 1989) would be the most valid, because it attempts to diagnose women who have relatively asymptomatic follicular phases and severely symptomatic luteal phases.

Contrary to our expectations, the absolute severity method did not consistently yield the most homogeneous LLPDD and non-LLPDD groups. Of the three scoring methods, it produced cases with the most symptomatic luteal phases, but all methods yielded cases with comparably low follicular phase symptomatology. Both the absolute severity and the percent change methods produced the expected finding that women with LLPDD were younger than women who did not meet the criteria of these methods, but there were no other differences in demographic characteristics among groups defined by any method. More surprising was the relative lack of differences between LLPDD and non-LLPDD groups in psychiatric history, and especially in the likelihood of current psychiatric disorder. As in our previous analyses, in which slightly more cases were used than in this data set (Hurt et al. 1992), LLPDD diagnosed by effect size was related to an increased likelihood of past psychiatric disorder. Extending this finding, we observed an increased likelihood of mood disorder in the past only among women with LLPDD according to the effect size method.

We also examined the homogeneity of diagnostic groups created by aggregating the groups defined by the initial scoring methods. Our procedure, which is roughly comparable to that used by Hammarbäck and colleagues (1989) to distinguish what they termed "pure PMS" from "PMS aggravation," failed, like the single scoring methods, to produce marked differences between LLPDD and non-LLPDD groups in either demographic or psychiatric variables. Once again, however, there were large differences between the aggregate diagnostic groups in symptom reports. Women with LLPDD by the criteria of the change and the absolute severity methods were more severely symptomatic in the luteal phase than women with LLPDD by the change methods only, although the two groups were comparable in follicular phase symptoms.

Other investigators have observed that the methods currently used to diagnose PMS and LLPDD do not agree about what does and does not constitute a case (Gallant et al. 1992; Hurt et al. 1992; Metcalf et al. 1989; Schnurr 1989a). Our findings suggest that women who meet criteria for LLPDD are relatively homogeneous in their psychiatric and demographic status, regardless of the method used to score symptoms. What is troubling, however, is the failure of the methods we used to produce clear and consistent differences between women with and without LLPDD. A possible interpretation for this failure is that LLPDD is not a valid diagnostic category. We think that such a conclusion is premature. A plausible alternative explanation is Type II error, that is, that the general lack of differences we observed resulted from problems that obscured actual differences. These problems need to be solved before the validity of LLPDD can be determined.

One problem highlighted here is the inconsistency in symptom patterns demonstrated by many women over consecutive menstrual cycles. Like others (e.g., Ekholm 1991; Schnurr 1989a; Shaver and Woods 1985), we found that some women are inconsistently symptomatic. Our analyses raise questions about the practice of treating women who meet diagnostic criteria for LLPDD in only one of two cycles as though they are the same as women who show no evidence of LLPDD. We would propose that these women be separated from women who consistently do not meet diagnostic criteria. We found that doing so significantly enhanced the distinctiveness of the LLPDD group defined by effect size in terms of psychiatric history. In fact, once the women who met diagnostic criteria for LLPDD in only one of two cycles were removed from the non-LLPDD group, women with LLPDD according to the effect size method showed the decreased likelihood of current psychiatric disorder that we had expected for all LLPDD groups.

Another methodological problem that needs to be addressed before we can determine the diagnostic validity of LLPDD is how to ensure that symptoms in the luteal phase are not "merely an exacerbation of the symptoms of another disorder" (American Psychiatric Association 1987, p. 369). We had expected that the absolute severity scoring method would do so, because it is distinctive among the many existing scoring methods for diagnosing PMS or LLPDD in its intent to meet this requirement; the exception is Hammarbäck and colleagues' (1989) two-stage procedure for diagnosing PMS. The absolute severity method did not perform as expected because it, like the other scoring methods, allowed some women with relatively high follicular phase symptoms to receive a diagnosis; these women, in turn, were more likely than those with lower follicular phase scores to have a current psychiatric disorder. When we arbitrarily divided women with LLPDD according to each method on the basis of a simple rule for scoring follicular phase symptoms, we observed the expected decreased likelihood of current disorder in those with lower follicular phase symptomatology. Our success suggests that future work is needed to determine an optimal scoring procedure, for example, by signal detection methods (Schnurr 1989b) or other optimization strategies.

A third problem that needs to be addressed is how to determine functional impairment in women with LLPDD. This is not an issue of the scoring method used or the symptoms that are assessed, but rather, one involving the measurement of additional variables. None of the approaches currently used to diagnose either LLPDD or PMS specifically attempts to determine whether a given symptom interferes with occupational or social functioning. Recently, Gallant and colleagues (1992) reported the first detailed investigation of functional impairment over the menstrual cycle. They found that all women, especially those who provisionally (i.e., retrospectively) met criteria for LLPDD, reported luteal phase decreases in performance that were not corroborated by reports of the frequency of social and occupational problems. It would be tempting to conclude from these data that women with LLPDD are not functionally impaired. It is not possible to do so, however, because most of the women in the LLPDD group did not meet prospective diagnostic criteria according to a variety of scoring methods. What we can conclude is that functional impairment should be measured in future research on LLPDD. Our failure to include functional impairment in the diagnostic process of past studies means that we do not know how many women currently meet all of the DSM-III-R criteria for LLPDD.

Conclusions

To date, we do not know how many women meet the diagnostic criteria for LLPDD. If the functional impairment criterion is excluded, we know that 14%–45% of women who seek treatment for premenstrual symptoms will qualify for the diagnosis (Hurt et al. 1992). Our findings described in this chapter, along with studies reviewed in the subsequent chapters of this book, suggest some interesting biological and psychological alterations in these women that need further exploration in better-diagnosed samples.

After performing many analyses and attempting many variations of these analyses, we found no compelling evidence in favor of a single scoring method for the diagnosis of LLPDD. None of the scoring methods we used were consistently superior to the others in terms of maximizing diagnostic homogeneity. Instead, all had strengths and weaknesses. The primary effect of these methodological alternatives is to distinguish groups of women who differ in their cycle-related symptomatology. If LLPDD is a valid diagnostic entity, all of the methods used in our study need further refinement.

The complexities we have presented may be overwhelming to the clinician or researcher who wants to know how to diagnose LLPDD. We have shown that there are many methodological issues to consider in this process—including scoring methods, consistency, and distinguishing symptom occurrence from symptom exacerbation—but have not resolved the issues. The present absolute severity criteria (Eckerd et al. 1989) or change criteria (Rubinow and Roy-Byrne 1984; Schnurr 1988) by themselves are not optimal for diagnosing LLPDD. An absolute severity–like rule seems necessary, however, to define cases that have sufficiently symptomatic luteal phases and asymptomatic follicular phases. Coupled with a more continuously scaled change criterion, it could be a good way to define a procedure for implementation in both practice and research. We plan to use this data set to derive better scoring procedures and encourage others to do the same. Replication, especially in non-treatment-seeking women, would enhance the validity of our findings. In the meantime, we recommend that diagnostic procedures for LLPDD include a measure of change (e.g., percent change, effect size) and an absolute severity requirement that is stricter than that proposed by Eckerd and colleagues (e.g., allowing up to 2 days during the follicular phase during which symptoms may be present, even in mild form). A good alternative would be to apply the statistical logic behind the diagnostic procedure proposed by Bäckström's research group (Ekholm 1991; Hammarbäck et al. 1989) to the symptoms of LLPDD.

Our study illustrates how methodological decisions in the diagnosis of LLPDD can produce variations in the homogeneity of groups who do and who do not meet diagnostic criteria. It serves as a reminder of the fallibility inherent in the process of psychiatric diagnosis. This fallibility requires us to continually refine our diagnostic methods, not only for LLPDD, but for all diagnoses.

References

American Psychiatric Association: Diagnostic and Statistical Manual of Mental Disorders, 3rd Edition. Washington, DC, American Psychiatric Association, 1980

American Psychiatric Association: Diagnostic and Statistical Manual of Mental Disorders, 3rd Edition, Revised. Washington, DC, American Psychiatric Association, 1987

DeJong R, Rubinow DR, Roy-Byrne P, et al: Premenstrual mood disorder and psychiatric illness. Am J Psychiatry 142:1359–1361, 1985

Eckerd MB, Hurt SW, Severino SK: Late luteal phase dysphoric disorder: relationship to personality disorders. Journal of Personality Disorders 4:338–344, 1989

Ekholm UB: Premenstrual syndrome: a study of change in cyclicity, severity and sexuality (doctoral dissertation). Umeå, Sweden, Umeå University Medical Dissertations, 1991

Feighner J, Robins L, Guze SB, et al: Diagnostic criteria for use in psychiatric research. Arch Gen Psychiatry 26:168–171, 1972

Freeman E, Sondheimer SJ, Rickels K: Effects of medical history factors on symptom severity in women meeting criteria for premenstrual syndrome. Obstet Gynecol 72:236–239, 1988

Gallant SJ, Popiel DA, Hoffman DM, et al: Using daily ratings to confirm premenstrual syndrome/late luteal phase dysphoric disorder, II: what makes a "real" difference? Psychosom Med 54:167–181, 1992

Hammarbäck S, Bäckström T, MacGibbon-Taylor B: Diagnosis of premenstrual tension syndrome: description and evaluation of a procedure for diagnosis and differential diagnosis. Journal of Psychosomatic Obstetrics and Gynaecology 10:25–42, 1989

Hartmann L: Presidential address: reflections on humane values and biopsychosocial integration. Am J Psychiatry 149:1135–1141, 1992

Hurt SW, Schnurr PP, Severino SK, et al: Late luteal phase dysphoric disorder in 670 women evaluated for premenstrual complaints. Am J Psychiatry 149:525–530, 1992

Kirk RE: Experimental Design: Procedures for the Behavioral Sciences (2nd Edition). Belmont, CA, Brooks/Cole, 1982

Magos AL, Studd JWW: Assessment of menstrual cycle symptoms by trend analysis. Am J Obstet Gynecol 155:271–277, 1986

Metcalf MG, Livesey JH, Wells JE: Assessment of the significance and severity of premenstrual tension, II: comparison of methods. J Psychosom Res 33:282–292, 1989

Rubinow DR, Roy-Byrne P: Premenstrual syndromes: overview from a methodologic perspective. Am J Psychiatry 141:163–172, 1984

Sanders D, Warner P, Bäckström T, et al: Mood, sexuality, hormones and the menstrual cycle, I: changes in mood and physical state: description of subjects and method. Psychosom Med 45:487–501, 1983

Schnurr PP: Some correlates of prospectively defined premenstrual syndrome. Am J Psychiatry 145:491–494, 1988

Schnurr PP: Measuring amount of symptom change in the diagnosis of premenstrual syndrome. Psychological Assessment: J Consult Clin Psychol 1:277–283, 1989a

Schnurr PP: Quantification of premenstrual symptom change: issues and methods. Paper presented at the National Institute of Mental Health/National Institute of Child Health and Human Development Workshop on LLPDD: New Research Directions. Washington, DC, NIMH/NICHHD, October 4, 1989b

Shaver JF, Woods N: Concordance of perimenstrual symptoms across two cycles. Res Nurs Health 8:313–319, 1985

Stout A, Steege JF, Blazer DG, et al: Comparison of lifetime psychiatric diagnoses in premenstrual syndrome clinic and community samples. J Nerv Ment Dis 174:517–522, 1986

West CP: The characteristics of 100 women presenting to a gynecological clinic with premenstrual complaints. Acta Obstet Gynecol Scand 68:743–747, 1989

℘ 3 ℘

Biological Correlates of Premenstrual Complaints

Barbara L. Parry, M.D.

The biomedical model is disease oriented, not patient oriented.

Engel 1979, p. 158

Historically, many theories have been proposed for the etiology of premenstrual dysphoria. This chapter reviews the evidence for biological etiologies. The studies selected for review include those that document prospective ratings of symptoms, use control groups, and have been published within the last 5 years. Particularly important or controversial studies that may not have included all the aforementioned criteria are also discussed. By means of this literature review, it is hoped that the reader may gain further understanding of the potential biological substrate that may predispose certain vulnerable women to dysphoric mood changes. The chapter is divided into six biological categories: 1) gonadal steroids and gonadotropins, 2) neurovegetative signs (sleep, appetite changes), 3) neuroendocrine factors, 4) serotonin and other neurotransmitters, 5) β-endorphin, and 6) other potential substrates (including prostaglandins, vitamins, electrolytes, and CO_2).

Gonadal Steroids and Gonadotropins

Rubinow and colleagues (1988) examined estradiol, progesterone, follicle-stimulating hormone (FSH), luteinizing hormone (LH), testosterone-estradiol–binding globulin, dehydroepiandrosterone sulfate, dehydrotestosterone, prolactin, and cortisol in 17 women with prospectively confirmed premenstrual syndrome (PMS) and 9 control subjects. PMS had been diagnosed according to daily ratings recorded by the subjects for two cycles and according to criteria requiring a 30% increase in the mean ratings recorded during the follicular phase compared with the luteal phase. Blood samples were drawn at 8:00 A.M. during the early, mid-, and late follicular phases and the early, mid-, and late luteal phases of the menstrual cycle. No diagnosis-related changes were found in any of the hormones. The authors suggested the need for dynamic rather than baseline measures to examine biological differences in women with PMS.

Hammarbäck and colleagues (1989) examined 18 women with PMS (no control subjects) who had been diagnosed according to daily ratings recorded for two cycles. Blood samples for estradiol, progesterone, FSH, and LH were taken daily during the luteal phase. Increased estradiol and progesterone levels were associated with increased symptomatology. Increased FSH levels were inversely related to symptoms of breast swelling and tenderness. The authors suggested that the relationship among estradiol, progesterone, and FSH may be important in the production of PMS symptoms.

Watts and colleagues (1985) measured levels of estradiol, progesterone, FSH, LH, cortisol, prolactin, thyroid-stimulating hormone (TSH), and testosterone in control subjects and 35 women with PMS who had been diagnosed by daily prospective ratings recorded for 2 months. Daily blood samples were taken between 8:30 A.M. and 5:00 P.M. (the study did not control for possible circadian variation) during weeks 1–4 of the menstrual cycle. Ovulation was determined by ultrasound. Women with PMS were found to have earlier time of ovulation, possibly a longer luteal phase, and increased cortisol levels. Although there was some suggestion that estradiol levels peaked earlier in women with PMS compared with control subjects, there were no differences in the levels of these and other measured hormones between the two groups. In contrast, Ying and colleagues (1987) examined a group of 83 infertile women undergoing timed endometrial biopsy for the assessment of luteal phase adequacy. Their data suggested that the hormonal milieu associated with luteal phase defects did not correlate with premenstrual symptoms.

Halbreich and colleagues (1986) examined the rate of change of gonadal hormones in relationship to PMS symptomatology. A total of 17 women with PMS that had been prospectively confirmed according to daily ratings and the Premenstrual Assessment Form (Endicott et al. 1986) and 3 control subjects had blood levels drawn between 8:00 A.M. and 10:00 A.M. every other day to determine estradiol and progesterone levels. Clinical assessment was used to identify the most symptomatic and the least symptomatic individuals. A faster rate of change of progesterone levels was associated with more severe symptomatology, with a time lag of 4–7 days between the hormonal increase or decrease and the appearance of symptoms in women with PMS. As noted, however, only three control subjects were studied.

Bäckström and colleagues (1985) studied seven women with PMS diagnosed according to 1 month of daily prospective ratings and seven control subjects who had undergone hysterectomy. The methods of these authors included enucleation of the corpus luteum. The luteal phase in women with PMS was associated with decreased levels of progesterone and FSH and increased levels of estradiol. The authors suggested that these findings may implicate increased inhibin levels in women with PMS. Many of the women had uterine fibroids and other medical reasons for hysterectomy. Because of the difficulty of performing the techniques used in that study, it has not been replicated.

Many investigators believe that there may be underlying biological vulnerabilities in women with PMS that may be triggered by changes in reproductive hormones. To date, however, there is insufficient evidence that estrogen or progesterone alone is the sole cause of PMS. One strategy being used to address this question is to suppress the hypothalamic-gonadal axis with gonadotropin-releasing hormone and then replace gonadal hormones in different dosages. These studies are still in a preliminary stage. In a study by Mortola and colleagues (1991), gonadotropin-releasing hormone agonist seemed to reduce symptoms concomitant with inducing amenorrhea, but the addition of estrogen and progesterone had equivocal results.

In another important study by Schmidt and colleagues (1991), women with late luteal phase dysphoric disorder (LLPDD) were given a progesterone antagonist, mifepristone (RU-486), to induce early menses in the mid-luteal phase. To another group of similar women they gave mifepristone plus human chorionic gonadotropin to preserve ovarian function. A third group received placebo. Despite the alteration of the endocrine phases of the menstrual cycle by this method, the timing and severity of symptoms were similar in the three groups. Neither the blockage of progesterone alone nor the truncations of the luteal phase altered the course or severity of symptoms. The results of this study suggest that PMS symptoms are not due only to the endocrine events occurring during the late luteal phase of the menstrual cycle. They also suggest that premenstrual symptoms could not be attributed only to psychological factors arising from anticipation of menstruation among women. In other words, the study indicated what PMS is not; it did not indicate what PMS is.

Summary

Although several studies have been suggestive of differences in the pattern of estrogen and progesterone secretion in women with PMS and control subjects, many other studies have not found differences, and no consistent or identifiable pattern has been established that can differentiate women with PMS from control subjects. The work of Hammarbäck and colleagues (1989, 1991) suggests that spontaneous anovulatory cycles cause the disappearance of cyclical symptoms in women with PMS. It may be, then, that it is the indirect effect of ovarian steroids in relation to other neurotransmitter, neuroendocrine, or circadian systems that precipitates premenstrual mood changes, rather than simply the direct effects of the increased or decreased levels of these steroid hormones. Studies of women who have undergone hysterectomy, however, support the effect of expectation bias on the appearance of symptoms (Metcalf et al. 1991).

Neurovegetative Signs and Psychophysiological Responses

Both-Orthman and colleagues (1988) examined appetite changes in 21 women with PMS that had been diagnosed by 3 months of daily self-ratings and 13 control subjects confirmed as not having PMS by 2 months of daily ratings. In women with PMS, increased appetite on the Premenstrual Assessment Form correlated with depressed mood. These findings led the authors to suggest links between PMS and atypical depressions and to implicate the possible role of the serotonin neurotransmitter system.

Mauri and colleagues (1988) examined self-reports of sleep during the premenstrual phase in 14 women with PMS that had been diagnosed with prospective assessments and 26 control subjects. Their methods also included two retrospective questionnaires, the Post-Sleep Inventory (Webb et al. 1976) and the Premenstrual Tension Syndrome form of Steiner (a yes/no questionnaire [Steiner et al. 1980]). Women with PMS reported increased sleep disturbances during the luteal phase. Sleep disturbances were used to differentiate between women with PMS and control subjects with 82% accuracy. The questionnaires, however, were based on subjective, retrospective reports.

Parry and colleagues (1989) measured sleep electroencephalography results, temperature, and wrist movement activity during the menstrual cycle in eight women with PMS and eight control subjects who had been screened using 2 months of daily ratings and weekly ratings using the Hamilton Rating Scale for Depression (Hamilton 1960) and the Beck Depression Inventory (Beck et al. 1979). Sleep electroencephalography recordings were made twice weekly for the duration of one menstrual cycle. Activity was measured daily using a wrist activity monitor, and temperature was measured by means of a nocturnal indwelling rectal probe. Women with PMS had more Stage II sleep and less rapid-eye-movement sleep than control subjects. There were no significant differences between the groups with regard to daily wrist activity measurements. Women with PMS had an earlier minimum nocturnal temperature than control subjects at all phases of the menstrual cycle, but the differences were not statistically significant. Both groups had increased awakenings during the late luteal phase. The sleep changes in women with PMS, though different from those in control subjects, did not parallel the sleep changes characteristic of women with major depressive disorders.

More recently, Lee and colleagues (1990) examined sleep changes in healthy women during the follicular and luteal phases. In women reporting more negative symptoms premenstrually on the Profile of Mood States (McNair et al. 1971; subjects were not evaluated for LLPDD a priori), there was an associated decrease of delta-wave sleep.

Van den Akker and Steptoe (1989) examined psychophysiological responses (heart rate, skin conductance, and electromyography results) in 16 women reporting severe premenstrual symptoms and in 8 control subjects but found no marked differences in resting autonomic activity.

Summary

These studies provide pilot data that suggest some differences in neurovegetative signs and symptoms (sleep and appetite) during the menstrual cycle in women with PMS and control subjects. The rationale for further investigation of these findings is discussed in Chapter 11.

Neuroendocrine Factors

Thyroid Hormone

Brayshaw and Brayshaw (1987), in a very controversial study in which retrospective questionnaires were used, identified 20 women with and 12 women without PMS. The authors performed thyroid-releasing hormone (TRH) infusions and then treated symptomatic women with levothyroxine (Synthroid). They claimed that women with PMS showed increased TSH responses to TRH and that 100% of the women with PMS responded to levothyroxine. The study has been criticized because the women with PMS were not diagnosed according to prospective ratings; the subject population included women who had thyroid disorder, affective disorder, and anorexia, but not PMS; and there were no outcome measures.

In contrast, Roy-Byrne and colleagues (1987) found no group or follicular-luteal phase differences in TSH and prolactin levels after TRH infusion in 14 women with prospectively confirmed PMS and control subjects (documented by daily ratings and 30% change criteria). They did, however, report increased variability of TSH responses to TRH (blunted and augmented responses) in symptomatic women compared with control subjects.

Casper and colleagues (1989) also found no differences in TSH or prolactin response to TRH during either the follicular or the luteal phases in 15 women with PMS and 19 control subjects. Subjects for this study had been selected according to ratings of visual analog scales recorded every third day for one (control subjects) to two (PMS subjects) cycles.

More recently, Nikolai and colleagues (1990) studied baseline thyroid function (thyroxine, triiodothyronine uptake, triiodothyronine, TSH, and TSH response to TRH) in 15 control subjects and 44 women with PMS that had been diagnosed by daily diaries, using the scoring system of Abraham (1983). The results showed no significant thyroid disease in women with PMS and that levothyroxine was no better than placebo in the treatment of PMS.

Prolactin

Parry and colleagues (1991) found that, in eight women with PMS who completed daily ratings for several cycles, there were normal TSH responses but enhanced prolactin responses to TRH administered during the follicular and luteal phases. In addition, in this study, cerebrospinal fluid (CSF) samples for 3-methoxy–4-hydroxyphenylglycol (MHPG), homovanillic acid, 5-hydroxyindoleacetic acid, β-endorphin, γ-aminobutyric acid, and prostaglandins were obtained from women with PMS during an asymptomatic follicular phase and a symptomatic luteal phase. MHPG levels in CSF were significantly higher during the premenstrual phase than during the follicular phase. Follicular and luteal phase dexamethasone suppression tests were performed in subsequent months after initial circadian hormone profiles of cortisol were obtained. Baseline cortisol levels showed significant increases during the late follicular phase, which was probably an effect of estrogen. Most (62%) of the women showed nonsuppression to dexamethasone. However, this abnormality occurred during both the follicular and luteal phases of the menstrual cycle.

Cortisol

Other groups have examined differences in cortisol levels in women with PMS and in control subjects. Haskett and colleagues (1984) examined urinary free cortisol and dexamethasone suppression test results in women with PMS. Forty-two women with PMS were selected on the basis of self-reports and clinical interviews during the follicular and luteal phases (no daily ratings, no control subjects). A 1-mg dexamethasone suppression test was administered, and levels of urinary free cortisol (24 hours) were obtained on cycle days 9 and 26. There was no cortisol hypersecretion, and there was normal suppression of cortisol levels after the dexamethasone suppression test was administered. No changes were found in urinary free cortisol levels during the follicular and luteal phases. The authors suggest that PMS is not a model for endogenous depression.

Roy-Byrne and colleagues (1986) also examined dexamethasone suppression test results in 11 women with PMS that had been prospectively confirmed by daily ratings that were recorded for 2 months. No differences in dexamethasone suppression test results during the follicular and luteal phases were found either in women with PMS or in control subjects.

Steiner and colleagues (1984) examined the circadian profile of prolactin, growth hormone, and cortisol levels in two women with PMS and two control subjects assessed by Moos's (1968) Menstrual Distress Questionnaire. Blood samples were obtained every 30 minutes for 24 hours during the follicular and luteal phases. Increased prolactin levels were found during the luteal phase in both women with PMS and control subjects (normal growth hormone and cortisol). The small sample size, however, limits the degree to which the findings can be generalized.

Glucose

Reid and colleagues (1986) examined oral glucose tolerance by administration of a 5-hour glucose tolerance test in six women with PMS (assessed by Steiner and colleagues' [1980] Premenstrual Tension Questionnaire, not daily ratings) and five control subjects. Glucose tolerance did not differ between the follicular and luteal phases or between control subjects and women with PMS. In addition, there were no differences in glucose, insulin, or glucagon responses to naloxone. Denicoff and colleagues (1990) also examined the results of glucose tolerance tests in 11 women with prospectively confirmed PMS during the follicular and luteal phases. Although the women experienced hypoglycemic symptoms, the symptoms were not specific to the luteal phase and did not resemble the subjects' PMS symptoms.

Diamond and colleagues (1989) performed hyperglycemic clamp studies in control subjects during the mid-follicular and mid-luteal phases of the menstrual cycle and found that glucose metabolism was impaired during the luteal phase, an effect that could not be explained by differences in the plasma insulin response. However, these subjects were not selected or screened for menstrual cycle–related mood changes.

Melatonin

Parry and colleagues (1990) examined the melatonin circadian profile in eight women with PMS (documented by 2 months of daily ratings) and eight age-matched control subjects during the early follicular, late follicular, mid-luteal, and late luteal phases. Women with PMS showed significantly lower levels of melatonin than control subjects and a significant earlier offset of the melatonin secretion at all phases of the menstrual cycle. These findings suggest chronobiologic disturbances in women with PMS.

Summary

Although a variety of differences in neuroendocrine systems have been reported, there are no consistent findings with respect to thyroid, cortisol, prolactin, or glucose abnormalities in women with PMS compared with control subjects. Melatonin secretion in women with PMS and control subjects appears to be different, but the findings have yet to be replicated.

Serotonin and Other Neurotransmitter Systems

Ashby and colleagues (1988) examined alterations of serotonergic mechanisms and monoamine oxidase in women with PMS (sample size not described) that had been diagnosed according to daily visual analog scales for anxiety for two menstrual cycles. The criteria used in this study required a 30% increase in the mean ratings recorded during the follicular phase compared with the luteal phase. Blood samples were obtained premenstrually (days −1 to −9) and postmenstrually (days 5–9) for platelet uptake and content of 5-hydroxytryptophan, monoamine oxidase, and tryptophan. The V_{max} (concentration) of 5-hydroxytryptophan uptake and content was lower premenstrually in women with PMS than in control subjects. Monoamine oxidase concentrations were lower postmenstrually than premenstrually. There were no significant changes in tryptophan concentrations. This study focused only on women with PMS anxiety. The findings suggest that serotonergic circadian rhythms play a role in PMS. A follow-up report by Ashby and colleagues (1990) indicated that plasma obtained from women with PMS caused less stimulation of 5-hydroxytryptophan uptake than did plasma from control subjects.

Taylor and colleagues (1984) also examined serotonin levels and platelet uptake in 16 women with PMS who had been assessed by the Menstrual Distress Questionnaire (Moos 1968). Blood levels were drawn during the premenstrual and postmenstrual phases. The V_{max} of serotonin was significantly lower during the premenstrual phase. There were no differences in K_m (affinity) values. The study used no control subjects, the screening of subjects was not described, and the cycle phase was not documented. However, the findings are consistent with those of Ashby and colleagues (1988).

Rapkin and colleagues (1987) examined serotonin levels in whole blood in 14 women with PMS and 13 age-matched control subjects. Subjects were selected according to symptom diaries kept for 1 month, results of the Profile of Mood States (McNair et al. 1971), and the 30% criteria described previously in this chapter. Blood samples were obtained during the late luteal and premenstrual phases. Serotonin levels in women with PMS were lower during the last 10 days of the cycle. Although the time of day at which samples were collected was not specified and diaries were obtained for only 1 month, this was otherwise a methodologically sound study.

Malmgren and colleagues (1987) examined platelet serotonin uptake and vitamin B_6 treatment in 19 women with PMS and 19 age-matched control subjects who completed the Menstrual Distress Questionnaire (Moos 1968) and Spielberger and colleagues (1970) anxiety questionnaires on cycle days 5–7 and 25–27. Blood samples were obtained during the premenstrual and postmenstrual phases. There were no differences in platelet serotonin uptake in the two groups: lower V_{max} values occurred in the spring. This study has been criticized for not obtaining daily symptom ratings.

Uriel Halbreich (personal communication, December 1988) reported that in women seeking treatment for dysphoric premenstrual changes (prospectively evaluated), the pharmacokinetic disposition of tryptophan was unchanged during the menstrual cycle. He observed a premenstrual blunting in the responses of prolactin and cortisol to an 8-g tryptophan loading dose, which suggests a role for the serotonergic system in the formation of symptoms.

Rojansky and colleagues (1991) reported that imipramine receptor binding was lower in prospectively evaluated women with dysphoric premenstrual changes than in control subjects during the early luteal phase. Although there was no consistent change from the asymptomatic early luteal phase to the symptomatic late luteal phase, the authors suggested that a preexisting vulnerability to the development of premenstrual dysphoric changes might be related to impaired gonadal hormone modulation of the serotonergic system.

In addition to the CSF studies of dopamine, serotonin, and norepinephrine reported by Parry and colleagues (see "Neuroendocrine Factors" in this chapter), in which an increase in MHPG levels in CSF was found premenstrually in women with PMS, Uriel Halbreich (personal communication, December 1991) reported higher numbers of α_2-adrenergic receptors in women with dysphoric PMS during the follicular phase, and even more so during the late luteal phase, than in control subjects.

In previous studies, Schrijver and colleagues (1987) reported higher rates of urinary MHPG excretion in women with PMS than in control subjects, and DeLeon-Jones and colleagues (1982) reported downregulation of premenstrual urinary MHPG with therapeutic lithium treatment.

Summary

With the exception of the study by Malmgren and colleagues (1987), in which daily ratings were not obtained, the studies of serotonin levels in women with PMS compared with control subjects showed a consistent decrease in the V_{max} or levels of serotonin premenstrually. Studies with large sample sizes in well-diagnosed women with PMS and control subjects are needed to replicate these findings, but the results to date show a consistent trend. Given that melatonin is synthesized from serotonin, these data are consistent with the previously reported data on melatonin (see "Neuroendocrine Factors" in this chapter). Some preliminary data from CSF studies (Parry et al. 1991) and urinary and plasma studies (DeLeon-Jones et al. 1982; U. Halbreich, unpublished data, December 1991; Schrijver et al. 1987) suggest a role for the noradrenergic system.

β-Endorphin

Chuong and colleagues (1985) examined neuropeptide levels in 20 women with PMS and 20 control subjects. Women with PMS completed daily diaries and the Menstrual Distress Questionnaire (Moos 1968) for 3 months, and control subjects completed daily diaries and the Menstrual Distress Questionnaire for 1 month. Blood samples were collected every 2–3 days for 1 month for β-endorphin. β-Endorphin levels were lower in women with PMS than in control subjects. In women with PMS, levels measured during the luteal phase were lower than those measured during the follicular phase. There were no changes in neurotensin, human pancreatic peptide, vasointestinal peptide, gastrin, or bombesin levels. The authors suggested that, although peripheral measures were taken, β-endorphin levels may be a marker for the premenstrual state (circadian effects were not taken into account).

Facchinetti and colleagues (1987) also examined plasma β-endorphin levels in 11 women with PMS and 8 control subjects who completed the Menstrual Distress Questionnaire (Moos 1968) every 2 days. Blood samples were collected every 2–3 days for 1 month to determine levels of β-endorphin and β-lipotropin. Women with PMS showed a decrease in β-endorphin levels before and during menses. Normal values were obtained in these women during the follicular phase. No changes were observed in control subjects, and no changes in β-lipotropin levels were observed during the menstrual cycle. Although there were no daily ratings, the investigators carried out prospective assessments with the Menstrual Distress Questionnaire every other day. The authors implicate the failure of central opioid tonus premenstrually.

Tulenheimo and colleagues (1987) examined plasma β-endorphin immunoreactivity in 12 women with premenstrual tension who had been diagnosed with daily records (0–3 severity) and 14 control subjects. Morning blood samples were collected during the mid- and late follicular phases, the early and late luteal phases, and the premenstrual cycle phase. (The authors did not define the difference between the late luteal phase and the premenstrual phase in their study.) β-Endorphin levels were lower in women with premenstrual tension than in control subjects during the early luteal phase. In the women with premenstrual tension, there were no significant differences in β-endorphin levels during the follicular and luteal phases.

Summary

Although differences in assay sensitivity and circadian variability need to be accounted for, the studies consistently show that plasma β-endorphin levels are lower in women with PMS than in control subjects during the luteal phase. Measures of β-endorphin in CSF of women with PMS do not decline premenstrually (Parry et al. 1991). Since β-endorphin is a peptide released into portal circulation through the pituitary gland, the fact that differences are found peripherally is interesting, even though it may not be readily inferred that PMS is caused by decreases in β-endorphin acting on the central nervous system.

Other Potential Substrates

Jakubowicz and colleagues (1984) examined prostaglandins in women with PMS who were treated with mefenamic acid. Although 80 women were treated with mefenamic acid, only 19 were selected (according to a daily symptom checklist kept for one cycle) to participate in a 3-month, double-blind, crossover trial. Blood samples were obtained every 3 days. Although 86% of women improved when administered mefenamic acid, 500 mg three times daily, versus placebo, there were no changes in prostaglandin levels during the menstrual cycle, and prostaglandin levels were lower in women with PMS than in control subjects.

Mira and colleagues (1988) examined vitamins and trace elements in women with PMS. Thirty-eight women with PMS and 23 control subjects completed prospective symptom reports for three cycles. Samples were collected during the mid-follicular and premenstrual cycle phases for magnesium, zinc, and vitamins A, E, and B$_6$. No differences between groups were found during the cycle for any of the nutritional parameters.

Chuong and colleagues (1990) examined vitamin A levels in 10 women with PMS and 10 control subjects, diagnosed using daily dairies, at 2- to 3-day intervals throughout three menstrual cycles. No significant changes were noted between the control subjects and the women with PMS during either the luteal or the follicular phase.

Varma (1984) examined hormones and electrolytes in 25 women with PMS and 10 control subjects who had been selected by daily visual analog scales. Blood samples were obtained on days 3, 7, 11, 15, 19, 24, and 27 of each cycle. No differences in sodium or potassium levels were found in the women with PMS and control subjects, and there were no differences seen among phases of the menstrual cycle. Although there was a slight increase in cortisol levels during the luteal phase in the women with the most severe cases of PMS, levels were still in the normal range. No differences between the groups were found for estradiol, progesterone (slight increase in estrogen-to-progesterone ratio in women with PMS in the luteal phase), prolactin, FSH, or LH.

Rojansky and Halbreich (1991) examined the severity of symptoms and hormonal correlates in 78 sterilized (via tubal ligation) and nonsterilized women with prospectively confirmed PMS. No significant differences could be demonstrated between the groups. The authors concluded that premenstrual symptoms are not associated with tubal sterilization.

Harrison and colleagues (1989) found women with LLPDD to be more sensitive to the anxiolytic properties of CO_2 inhalation (double-breath or rebreathing) and lactate infusion than asymptomatic control subjects. In their study, none of the control subjects developed intense anxiety or panic attacks, whereas over half of the women with LLPDD did so. These findings suggest that women with LLPDD and anxiety disorders may have a shared vulnerability.

Summary

The studies do not support prostaglandin, nutritional (vitamin), or electrolyte disturbances in women with PMS. The work regarding CO_2 inhalation suggests biological differences between women with LLPDD and control subjects and perhaps a shared vulnerability of women with LLPDD and those with anxiety or panic disorders.

Conclusions

It is apparent that further biological differences among women with premenstrual affective, cognitive, and behavioral symptomatology cannot be deciphered without close attention to the diagnostic procedures used for subject selection in the different studies. The lack of standardized procedures for diagnosis is the rate-limiting factor in furthering the search for biological differences in these individuals. Studies in which certain systems are examined cannot be compared if different groups use variable selection criteria for their subjects. Thus, the first step in the exploration of the biological vulnerabilities that predispose women to severe premenstrual mood disturbances is to develop standardized diagnostic criteria so as to enhance sample homogeneity.

My hypothesis, generated from interpretations and conclusions drawn from reviewing studies on biological differences in women with premenstrual mood disorders compared with control subjects, is that there exists in women with PMS a biological vulnerability, manifested most readily in the serotonergic and melatonin systems (with possible contributions from the noradrenergic system), that is unmasked premenstrually. Like the postpartum period for affective illness, the threshold for presentation or the protective factor against affective symptoms is lowered during the premenstrual phase because of the interaction of the altered hormonal milieus with neurotransmitter, neuroendocrine, and circadian systems. There is an altered response to steroid effects on the brain at this time because of a priori altered receptor substrate sensitivity.

References

Abraham GE: Nutritional factors in the etiology of the premenstrual tension syndrome. J Reprod Med 28:446–464, 1983

Ashby CR, Carr LA, Cook CL, et al: Alteration of platelet serotonergic mechanisms and monoamine oxidase activity in premenstrual syndrome. Biol Psychiatry 24:225–233, 1988

Ashby CR, Carr LA, Cook CL, et al: Alteration of 5-HT uptake by plasma fractions in the premenstrual syndrome. J Neural Transm Gen Sect 79:41–50, 1990

Bäckström T, Smith S, Lothian H, et al: Prolonged follicular phase and depressed gonadotropins following hysterectomy and corpus luteectomy in women with premenstrual tension syndrome. Clin Endocrinol (Oxf) 22:723–732, 1985

Beck AT, Rush AJ, Shaw ES, et al: Cognitive Therapy of Depression. New York, Guilford, 1979

Both-Orthman B, Rubinow DR, Hoban C, et al: Menstrual cycle phase-related changes in appetite in patients with premenstrual syndrome and in control subjects. Am J Psychiatry 145:628–631, 1988

Brayshaw ND, Brayshaw DD: Premenstrual syndrome and thyroid dysfunction. Integrative Psychiatry 5:179–193, 1987

Casper RF, Patel-Christopher A, Powell AM: Thyrotropin and prolactin response to thyrotropin-releasing hormone in premenstrual syndrome. J Clin Endocrinol Metab 68:608–612, 1989

Chuong CJ, Coulam CB, Kao PC, et al: Neuropeptide levels in premenstrual syndrome. Fertil Steril 44:760–765, 1985

Chuong CJ, Dawson EB, Smith ER: Vitamin A levels in premenstrual syndrome. Fertil Steril 54:643–647, 1990

DeLeon-Jones FA, Val E, Herts C: MHPG excretion and lithium treatment during premenstrual tension syndrome: a case report. Am J Psychiatry 139:950–952, 1982

Denicoff KD, Hoban C, Grover GW, et al: Glucose tolerance testing in women with premenstrual syndrome. Am J Psychiatry 147:477–480, 1990

Diamond MP, Simonson DC, De Fronzo RA: Menstrual cyclicity has a profound effect on glucose homeostasis. Fertil Steril 52:204–208, 1989

Endicott J, Nee J, Cohen J, et al: Premenstrual changes: patterns and correlates of daily ratings. J Affect Disord 10:127–135, 1986

Engel GL: The biopsychosocial model and the education of health professionals. Gen Hosp Psychiatry 1:156–165, 1979

Facchinetti F, Martignoni E, Petraglia F, et al: Premenstrual fall of plasma β-endorphin in patients with premenstrual syndrome. Fertil Steril 47:570–573, 1987

Halbreich U, Endicott J, Goldstein S, et al: Premenstrual changes and changes in gonadal hormones. Acta Psychiatr Scand 74:576–586, 1986

Hamilton M: A rating scale for depression. J Neurol Neurosurg Psychiatry 23:56–62, 1960

Hammarbäck S, Damber JE, Bäckström T, et al: Relationship between symptoms severity and hormone changes in women with premenstrual syndrome. J Clin Endocrinol Metab 68:125–130, 1989

Hammarbäck S, Ekholm UB, Bäckström T: Spontaneous anovulation causing disappearance of cyclical symptoms in women with the premenstrual syndrome. Acta Endocrinol (Copenh) 125:132–137, 1991

Harrison WM, Sandberg D, Gorman JM, et al: Provocation of panic with carbon dioxide inhalation in patients with premenstrual dysphoria. Psychiatry Res 27:183–192, 1989

Haskett RF, Steiner M, Carroll BJ: A psychoendocrine study of premenstrual tension syndrome. J Affective Disord 6:191–199, 1984

Jakubowicz DL, Godard E, Dewhurst J: The treatment of premenstrual tension with mefenamic acid: analysis of prostaglandin concentrations. Br J Obstet Gynaecol 91:78–84, 1984

Lee KA, Shaver JF, Giblin EC, et al: Sleep patterns related to menstrual cycle phase and premenstrual affective symptoms. Sleep 13:403–409, 1990

Malmgren R, Collins A, Milsson CG: Platelet serotonin uptake and effects of vitamin B_6 treatment in premenstrual tension. Neuropsychobiology 18:83–88, 1987

Mauri M, Reid RL, MacLean AW: Sleep in the premenstrual phase: a self-report study of PMS patients and normal controls. Acta Psychiatr Scand 78:82–86, 1988

McNair DM, Lorr M, Pruppleman LF: Profile of Mood States. San Diego, CA, Educational and Industrial Testing Service, 1971

Metcalf MG, Livesey JH, Wells JE, et al: Premenstrual syndrome in hysterectomized women: mood and physical symptom cyclicity. J Psychosom Res 35:555–567, 1991

Mira M, Steward PM, Abraham SF: Vitamin and trace element status in premenstrual syndrome. Am J Clin Nutr 47:636–641, 1988

Moos RH: The development of a menstrual distress questionnaire. Psychosom Med 30:853–867, 1968

Mortola JF, Girton L, Fischer U: Successful treatment of severe premenstrual syndrome by combined use of gonadotropin-releasing hormone agonist and estrogen/progestin. J Clin Endocrinol Metab 71:252a–252f, 1991

Nikolai TF, Mulligan GM, Gribble RK, et al: Thyroid function and treatment in premenstrual syndrome. J Clin Endocrinol Metab 70:1108–1113, 1990

Parry BL, Mendelson WB, Duncan WC, et al: Longitudinal sleep EEG temperature and activity measurements across the menstrual cycle in patients with premenstrual depression and in age-matched controls. Psychiatry Res 30:285–303, 1989

Parry BL, Berga SL, Kripke DF, et al: Altered waveform of plasma nocturnal melatonin secretion in premenstrual depression. Arch Gen Psychiatry 47:1139–1146, 1990

Parry BL, Gerner RH, Wilkins JN, et al: CSF and neuroendocrine studies of premenstrual syndrome. Neuropsychopharmacology 5:127–137, 1991

Rapkin AJ, Edelmuth E, Chang LC, et al: Whole-blood serotonin in premenstrual syndrome. Obstet Gynecol 70:533–537, 1987

Reid RL, Greenaway-Coates A, Hahn PM, et al: Oral glucose tolerance during the menstrual cycle in normal women and women with alleged premenstrual "hypoglycemic" attacks: effects of naloxone. J Clin Endocrinol Metab 62:1167–1172, 1986

Rojansky N, Halbreich U: Prevalence and severity of premenstrual changes after tubal sterilization. J Reprod Med 36:551–555, 1991

Rojansky N, Halbreich U, Zander K, et al: Imipramine receptor binding and serotonin uptake in platelets of women with premenstrual changes. Gynecol Obstet Invest 31:146–152, 1991

Roy-Byrne PP, Rubinow DR, Qwirtsman H, et al: Cortisol response to dexamethasone in women with premenstrual syndrome. Neuropsychobiology 16:61–63, 1986

Roy-Byrne PP, Rubinow DR, Hoban C, et al: TSH and prolactin responses to TRH in patients with premenstrual syndrome. Am J Psychiatry 144:480–484, 1987

Rubinow DR, Hoban G, Grover GN, et al: Changes in plasma hormones across the menstrual cycle in patients with menstrually related mood disorders and in control subjects. Am J Obstet Gynecol 158:5–11, 1988

Schmidt PF, Nieman LK, Grover GN, et al: Lack of effect of induced menses on symptoms in women with premenstrual syndrome. N Engl J Med 324:1174–1179, 1991

Schrijver J, Louwerse ES, Bruinse HW, et al: Increased urinary MHPG excretion in premenstrual syndrome (PMS): the effect of vitamin B_6. Journal of Psychosomatic Obstetrics and Gynaecology 6:179–186, 1987

Spielberger CD, Gorsuch RL, Lushene RE: STAI Manual. Palo Alto, CA, Consulting Psychologists Press, 1970

Steiner M, Haskett RF, Carroll BJ: Premenstrual tension syndrome: the development of research diagnostic criteria and new rating scales. Acta Psychiatr Scand 62:177–190, 1980

Steiner M, Haskett RF, Carroll BJ: Circadian hormone secretory profiles in women with severe premenstrual tension syndrome. Br J Obstet Gynaecol 91:466–471, 1984

Taylor DL, Matthew RJ, Ho BT, et al: Serotonin levels and platelet uptake during premenstrual tension. Neuropsychobiology 12:16–18, 1984

Tulenheimo A, Laatkainen T, Salminen K: Plasma β-endorphin immunoreactivity in premenstrual tension. Br J Obstet Gynaecol 94:26–29, 1987

Van den Akker D, Steptoe D: Psychophysiological responses in women reporting severe premenstrual symptoms. Psychosom Med 51:319–328, 1989

Varma TR: Hormones and electrolytes in premenstrual syndrome. Int J Gynaecol Obstet 22:51–58, 1984

Watts JFF, Butt WR, Edwards LR, et al: Hormonal studies in women with premenstrual tension. Br J Obstet Gynaecol 92:247–255, 1985

Webb WB, Bonnet M, Blume G: A post-sleep inventory. Percept Mot Skills 43:987–993, 1976

Ying YK, Soto-Albors CE, Randolph JF, et al: Luteal phase defect and premenstrual syndrome in an infertile population. Obstet Gynecol 69:96–98, 1987

ॐ 4 ॐ

A Focus on 5-Hydroxytryptamine (Serotonin) and Psychopathology

Sally K. Severino, M.D.

> Nothing exists in isolation. Whether a cell or a person, every system is influenced by the configuration of the systems of which each is a part, that is, by its environment . . . neither the cell nor the person can be fully characterized as a dynamic system without characterizing the larger system(s) . . . of which it is a part.
>
> Engel 1980, p. 537

Given Parry's (Chapter 3) conclusion that a promising area of research about the etiology of affective symptoms in women is the serotonin system, it is worthwhile to review the work that has appeared in the literature regarding serotonin and psychopathology. Such a perspective can provide a framework to guide future efforts to understand how this system might be involved with premenstrual symptomatology.

5-Hydroxytryptamine (5-HT), a vasoconstrictor in serum, was given the name "serotonin" in 1948. Long before, it had been called many names, including "vasotonin" and "enteramine." Synthetic 5-HT was introduced in 1951. With the discovery of 5-HT in the brain, attention turned to the possible role of this neurotransmitter in mental illness (Gilman et al. 1985).

About 90% (10 mg) of 5-HT in humans is located in entero-chromaffin cells in the gastrointestinal tract, and most of the remainder is located in platelets and the central nervous system. Most is synthesized in situ from tryptophan (see Figure 4–1) and stored in granular sites (Gilman et al. 1985).

Within the central nervous system, the cell bodies of serotonergic neurons are found in and around the midline raphe nuclei of the brain stem; the projections of these cells are widely distributed throughout the brain and spinal cord. The serotonergic system is the most extensive monoaminergic system in the brain stem. The neurotransmitter is thought to affect mood, appetitive behaviors, sleep, and temperature and to influence the release of growth

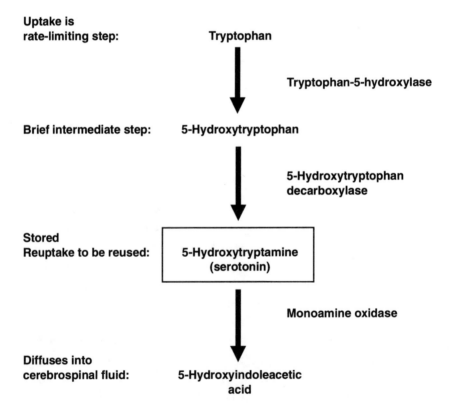

Figure 4–1. Metabolism of serotonin.

hormone, prolactin, luteinizing hormone, and follicle-stimulating hormone. In the pineal gland, serotonin serves as a precursor of the hormone melatonin (Gilman et al. 1985).

A circadian rhythm for 5-HT has been described in mice, rats, cats, lizards, and rabbits. Higher whole-brain levels have been found during or immediately before the animals' quiescent period (Gingras et al. 1990). The suprachiasmatic nucleus of the hypothalamus is the locus of a mammalian circadian pacemaker. The suprachiasmatic nucleus, which is usually synchronized to the environmental photoperiod, receives a large serotonergic projection from the raphe nuclei (Moore 1990). The question has arisen, then, of whether 5-HT can modulate the suprachiasmatic nucleus pacemaker.

Some evidence suggests that serotonin agonists can phase-shift the suprachiasmatic nucleus pacemaker in rats in vitro (Prosser et al. 1990). In vivo experiments in hamsters, however, have shown that serotonergic innervation is not necessary for circadian rhythmicity, although 5-HT may lend greater cohesiveness—that is, less variability—to circadian rhythms (Morin et al. 1990). In *Aplysia californica*, 5-HT, together with light, produces phase shifts in the ocular rhythm in a dose-dependent manner. Serotonin inhibits light-induced phase delays in ocular rhythm and enhances light-induced phase advances. Furthermore, the phase shifts produced when 5-HT is followed by light in the late night are larger than those produced by giving 5-HT and light simultaneously (Colwell 1990).

In humans, both dim and bright light augment 5-HT levels in blood throughout the day, whereas the effects of light on melatonin are less pronounced (Rao et al. 1990). There is some evidence that physiological, season-related changes in 5-HT uptake by platelets may be linked to the photoperiod, the maximal velocity of 5-HT uptake being higher in the spring and summer than in the autumn (Marazziti et al. 1990).

Results of studies in animals suggest sex-based differences in the responsivity of the 5-HT system and changes in 5-HT levels, depending on the phase of the estrous cycle (Fischette et al. 1984; McEwen and Parsons 1982). Attempts to alter serotonin turnover with estrogen and progesterone produced mixed results, perhaps because the time of day for administering the steroids was not controlled (McEwen and Parsons 1982).

Tam and colleagues (1985) prospectively studied six healthy women throughout three menstrual cycles, measuring mood and platelet 5-HT uptake on days 1, 10, and 24 at 9:30 A.M.. They found a significant linear rise of negative affect that occurred across each cycle and peaked on day 1. No significant correlation between mood scores and platelet uptake of 5-HT was found, however. Similarly, Ellis and colleagues (1992) studied platelet tritium-labeled imipramine binding in nine healthy women and found no significant relationship between maximal binding or dissociation constant and phase of the menstrual cycle, premenstrual symptoms, or estrogen or progesterone concentration. In another study of healthy women, the urinary metabolite of serotonin (5-hydroxyindoleacetic acid) was found to be highest during the follicular phase, lower during the luteal phase, and lowest during the premenstruum (de Tejada et al. 1978). Studies of steroid effects on 5-HT uptake, receptor systems of specific brain anatomical subdivisions, and the various mechanisms by which ovarian steroids can alter 5-HT receptors all need further elucidation.

More specifically, studies must clarify the effects of gonadal steroids on each of the steps in serotonin synthesis (see Figure 4–1), storage, release, and receptor activation. Steroid effects on tryptophan concentrations in plasma and brain, as well as on the transport of tryptophan into storage sites, also need clarification. Possible alterations in tryptophan-5-hydroxylase and tryptophan-5-hydroxylase decarboxylase by steroids affecting serotonin storage (in neurons), release, and reuptake must be determined. What, if any, effects do steroids produce on monoamine oxidase activity? What effects do steroids have on serotonin receptors ($5-HT_{1A}$, $5-HT_{1B}$, $5-HT_{1C}$, $5-HT_{1D}$, $5-HT_{1E}$, $5-HT_2$, $5-HT_{3A}$, $5-HT_{3B}$, $5-HT_{3C}$, $5-HT_4$), each of which is pharmacologically different? If behaviors are modulated by the interaction of serotonin receptors, in addition to being mediated by particular serotonin receptors (Glennon et al. 1991) and/or modified by the interaction of serotonin with other neurotransmitters (Awouters et al. 1990), how do gonadal hormones affect these receptor-receptor interactions? What effect does the environment have on serotonin levels (McGuire 1983)?

Serotonin and Premenstrual Syndrome/ Late Luteal Phase Dysphoric Disorder

Serotonin has been implicated as an etiological factor in premenstrual syndrome (PMS [Halbreich et al. 1991; Labrum 1983]), a condition characterized by mood and appetitive behaviors associated with monthly gonadal hormone changes.

Plasma Tryptophan

Two studies have addressed the question of tryptophan concentrations. Ashby and colleagues (1988) measured plasma tryptophan premenstrually (days −1 to −9) and postmenstrually (days 5–9) in women with PMS and found no significant changes. This is consistent with the findings of Odink and colleagues (1990). The latter group, in addition, found higher plasma levels of tryptophan in 19 women with PMS than in 19 control subjects across the entire menstrual cycle.

Tryptophan has been used to treat women with PMS, and the results have been mixed. One case report of the use of L-tryptophan alone for the treatment of PMS appears in the literature (Price et al. 1984–1985). The authors tried tryptophan in an effort to increase serotonin levels in one woman, on the premise that decreased serotonin levels could account for depression and other symptoms of PMS. The woman had experienced severe PMS for 11 years, since age 14, and had had both physical and psychological symptoms. It was the severity of the latter that brought her to the attention of the investigators, a team of psychiatrists. She was given tryptophan, 1,000 mg orally, 5 times daily. After 1 month, she still reported the physical symptoms, but her anxiety, depression, and tension levels had decreased, and she was sleeping better.

Harrison and colleagues (1984) tried tryptophan in combination with vitamin B_6 because it is intimately involved in the conversion of tryptophan to serotonin. Thirty physically healthy women who were between ages 21 and 42 and had been prospectively selected for PMS entered a single-blind, sequential study of placebo versus a combination of L-tryptophan and pyridoxine given throughout the entire menstrual cycle. All women were given placebo during the first treatment month. Those whose symptoms responded to placebo remained on placebo for the duration of the study. The other subjects ($n = 16$) were continued on 1.5 g of L-tryptophan combined with 50 mg of pyridoxine. These doses were doubled after each premenstrual phase during which there was no response, until maximum doses of 6.0 g of L-tryptophan plus 150 mg of pyridoxine were reached. Only six women received the maximum doses. Refusal to increase the dose occurred after the second dose level by women who reported daytime drowsiness, nausea, headaches, or overstimulation. Symptoms improved in only two of the women who completed the study. This improvement occurred at the second dose level of 3.0 g of L-tryptophan plus 100 mg of pyridoxine. The authors did not report the time of day at which treatments were administered, nor whether the doses were single or divided doses.

Blood Platelet Serotonin

Platelets have been used as a biological model of serotonergic presynaptic nerve endings (Stahl et al. 1982). In studies of women with PMS, Taylor and colleagues (1984) and Ashby and colleagues (1988) reported reduced platelet uptake of serotonin in women with PMS during the week before menstruation. Two subsequent reports, one by Ashby and colleagues (1990) and another by Steege and colleagues (1992), showed less serotonin uptake by platelets in women with PMS than in control subjects during both the follicular and luteal phases. The findings of Rapkin and colleagues (1987) lend further support for the finding of lower serotonin levels in women with PMS. They reported that whole-blood serotonin levels during the last 10 days of the menstrual cycle in 14 women with PMS were lower than those in 13 women without PMS. This study was methodologically sound, although the time of day at which samples were collected was not specified.

Rojansky and colleagues (1991) studied 18 women with and 9 women without PMS. They were ages 18–45, had been prospectively diagnosed, and were free of psychological or physical illness. Blood levels drawn at 9:00–10:00 A.M. at two menstrual cycle phases (early luteal and late luteal) were analyzed for 5-HT platelet uptake and imipramine binding. Subjects with PMS showed much interindividual variability with no consistent typical pattern or change related to the asymptomatic early luteal compared with the symptomatic late luteal phase. Their imipramine receptor binding, however, was lower than that in control subjects during the early luteal phase and was similar to that in control subjects in the late luteal phase. This study raises the question of to what degree age contributes to the interindividual variability. Perhaps studies should differentiate between women younger than age 30 years old and older than age 30 years (McBride et al. 1990).

Veeninga and Westenberg (1992) studied 38 women allegedly with and 18 women without late luteal phase dysphoric disorder (LLPDD). Women with LLPDD received 200 mg of L-5-hydroxytryptophan orally at 9:00 A.M. on day 26 and again 4 days after the beginning of the next menstrual cycle. Control subjects received this dosage on only one of those two days. Blood samples for cortisol, β-endorphin, 5-hydroxytryptophan, and 5-hydroxyindoleacetic acid were drawn just before the oral dose was given and again at every hour up to 4 hours after the dose was given. Platelet 5-hydroxytryptophan was also measured. The authors found no evidence of a role for serotonin in the pathophysiology of LLPDD. Their findings, however, must be evaluated in the context of the following aspects of the study design: 1) subjects with mental disorders were not excluded, 2) ratings of daily symptoms on only two menstrual cycle days were used to "confirm" the diagnosis of LLPDD without delineating the number of positive symptoms required or the impact of the symptoms on the women's ability to function, and 3) luteal and follicular phase blood samples were drawn from different menstrual cycles in the women with LLPDD and from only one menstrual cycle phase in the control subjects. These conclusions must therefore be regarded with caution.

Ashby and colleagues (1992) took their studies one step further. Rat forebrain synaptosomes were subjected to various amounts of plasma (10, 25, and 100 μl) obtained from six women with PMS and six control volunteers (ages 28–41 years) during both premenstrual and postmenstrual phases. The authors observed a volume-dependent decrease in the uptake of tritium-labeled 5-HT in synaptosomes in both groups at both phases of the menstrual cycle. Their results suggest that the plasma from all subjects contained endogenous substances that produced these effects. The plasma obtained premenstrually from the subjects with PMS produced greater inhibition than the plasma from the control subjects. This result raises the question of whether women with PMS have more endogenous substances or whether their endogenous substances are more active. Additionally, the plasma from control subjects produced significantly more inhibition of uptake during the postmenstrual phase than during the premenstrual phase; the plasma from the control subjects produced no difference in 5-HT uptake between phases. This suggests that control subjects possess a mechanism that mediates cyclic changes that may be lacking in women with PMS. This pilot study needs replication.

Neuroendocrine Challenge Tests

In a pilot study of women without PMS during the luteal phase of the menstrual cycle, Yatham and colleagues (1989) reported that the prolactin response to a buspirone challenge test was greater during the luteal phase, implying supersensitivity of the serotonin receptors. These researchers speculated that women with PMS may be even more sensitive. There is some preliminary evidence that there is a receptor component similar to 5-HT$_1$ demonstrated in the prolactin response to the buspirone challenge test (Coccaro et al. 1990).

In humans, changes in 5-HT function can be studied by measuring neuroendocrine responses to an infusion of the precursor for 5-HT, L-tryptophan. Normally, the challenge of an L-tryptophan infusion produces an increase in plasma prolactin and growth hormone. Bancroft and colleagues (1991) studied 13 women with and 13 women without premenstrual depression (prospectively determined) in the late luteal phase and the mid- to late follicular phase with the order of testing balanced. During both phases, the growth hormone response was lower in women with premenstrual depression than in control subjects. Similarly, the cortisol response was absent in women with premenstrual depression during both phases. The prolactin response to tryptophan was blunted premenstrually in both groups.

Moline and colleagues (1992) studied six women (ages 33–41 years) with PMS that had been diagnosed by 2 months of prospective daily ratings and two control women (ages 28 and 29 years). Each woman received a thyroid-releasing hormone challenge test (200 μg intravenously) during the follicular phase and late luteal phase of one menstrual cycle, followed by a fenfluramine challenge test (60 mg orally) during the follicular phase and late luteal phase of a subsequent menstrual cycle. Two women with PMS had abnormal responses to thyroid-releasing hormone and were excluded. There were no differences in the prolactin response of the remaining subjects to thyroid-releasing hormone, either between control and PMS groups or across the menstrual cycle in either group. The prolactin response to the fenfluramine challenge also did not differ between cycle phases in either group. The response to fenfluramine in the women with PMS, however, was significantly lower across the entire cycle than in the control women. In general, fenfluramine produces an increase in prolactin levels in human plasma that is believed to be mediated by the central serotonin system. This pilot study, therefore, suggests a difference between women with PMS and control subjects that involves the serotonin axis across the menstrual cycle.

Serotonin Agonists

Treatment of PMS with serotonergic drugs has been effective for some symptoms. Five serotonergic drugs have been reported to have efficacy in the treatment of PMS: buspirone, fluoxetine, D-fenfluramine, clomipramine, and fluvoxamine.

Although its mechanism of action is not clear, buspirone is known to bind with high affinity to serotonin (5-HT_{1A}) receptors (Huff and Dowd 1988). In the first clinical report of buspirone for PMS (an open trial), the drug ameliorated the symptoms of severe premenstrual anxiety in women diagnosed retrospectively with PMS (David et al. 1987). In a second pilot study, Rickels and colleagues (1989) assigned women with PMS to groups treated with either buspirone or placebo. (The methodology used to diagnose PMS in this study is unclear.) On a global scale, symptoms were significantly improved in women receiving buspirone. Individual symptoms such as depression and irritability, however, were not shown to be significantly improved in women receiving the drug over those receiving placebo.

More recently, fluoxetine, which inhibits neuronal serotonin uptake, was used in a placebo-controlled study (Rickels et al. 1990) and in three double-blind, randomized, placebo-controlled studies (Menkes et al. 1992; Stone et al. 1991; Wood et al. 1992). It was shown to be more effective than placebo for treating the affective symptoms of PMS/LLPDD.

Another serotonergic drug is D-fenfluramine, an appetite suppressant. It facilitates the release of serotonin from presynaptic nerve terminals and blocks its reuptake. In a double-blind crossover study of 17 overweight women with PMS, D-fenfluramine was shown to be more effective than placebo in suppressing appetite and improving mood during the luteal phase (Brzezinski et al. 1990; Wurtman 1990).

In a recent report (Sundblad et al. 1992), women with LLPDD received clomipramine, which is a serotonin reuptake inhibitor (25–75 mg; flexible doses), ($n = 20$) and placebo ($n = 20$). In all of three treatment cycles, clomipramine was significantly more effective than placebo in reducing premenstrual irritability and dysphoria in women with LLPDD.

One serotonin uptake blocker, fluvoxamine, was shown to be beneficial, but no better than placebo, in improving both somatic and affective symptoms in 20 women with premenstrual complaints (Veeninga et al. 1990). It should be noted that throughout the study, women rated symptoms on only 4 days of each menstrual cycle: days 4, 12, 22, and 26.

Serotonin Catabolism

Monoamine oxidase is the enzyme needed for the catabolism of serotonin (see Figure 4–1). Plasma monoamine oxidase activity has been reported to be significantly greater during the luteal phase than during the follicular phase of the menstrual cycle in regularly menstruating women (Briggs and Briggs 1972; Klaiber et al. 1971). Platelet monoamine oxidase activity, usually determined in blood drawn from fasting subjects, was found to peak during the ovulatory interval ($n = 13$ healthy women) and to be lowest 5–11 days later, during the luteal phase (Belmaker et al. 1974).

In a more recent study, platelet monoamine oxidase activity in women with PMS was compared with that in healthy control subjects (Hallman et al. 1987). The time of day that the platelets were drawn was not stated. Women with PMS ($n = 29$) had significantly lower platelet monoamine oxidase activity than the control subjects ($n = 20$). No variation in platelet monoamine oxidase activity was found throughout the menstrual cycle in either group of women, in contrast to the report of Belmaker and colleagues (1974). The findings of Hallman and colleagues (1987), however, are consistent with those of Feine and colleagues (1977), who found no significant variation in platelet monoamine oxidase activity throughout the menstrual cycle in 12 women with PMS.

Rapkin and colleagues (1988), on the other hand, were unable to find a difference in platelet monoamine oxidase B activity in women with PMS and in healthy control subjects. Diagnoses were made prospectively. The time of day that the platelets were drawn was not specified. These authors did not detect an effect due to menstrual cycle phase on enzyme activity, estradiol, or progesterone concentrations at any point throughout the menstrual cycle. They suggested that their work differed from that of others (e.g., Hallman et al. 1987) in subject selection and/or platelet isolation techniques.

Summary

Studies of serotonin in women with PMS/LLPDD compared with healthy control subjects show a consistent trend toward a decrease in the number of binding sites and levels of serotonin premenstrually (Eriksson et al. 1990). Some investigators hypothesize that LLPDD is a model of serotonin dysregulation (Lepage and Steiner 1991).

Serotonin and Eating Disorders

Because of the effect of serotonin on mood and appetitive behaviors, disturbed serotonin activity has been implicated in the development of eating disorders (Schreiber et al. 1991). Diets high in carbohydrates and low in protein increase brain serotonin in rats by facilitating the uptake of the precursor of serotonin—tryptophan—in the brain (Jimerson et al. 1990). Studies in healthy human subjects suggest that dieting can affect the neuroendocrine response to intravenous L-tryptophan in women but not in men (Goodwin et al. 1987). Clinical studies in humans with eating disorders have included studies of serotonin precursors and metabolites, as well as pharmacologic challenge studies. After careful review of the results of these studies, Jimerson and colleagues (1990) concluded that there was evidence for decreased central serotonin function that may influence the onset and persistence of binge eating in women with bulimia nervosa and women with anorexia nervosa who occasionally binge.

Plasma Tryptophan

No differences in concentrations of the essential amino acid precursor of serotonin—tryptophan—were found when the ratio of tryptophan to large neutral amino acids was measured in women of normal weight with bulimia nervosa ($n = 23$) and healthy control subjects ($n = 7$) and in depressed and nondepressed bulimic women (Lydiard et al. 1988). Changes in the ratio were found, however, when blood was sampled during the time that bulimic women were bingeing. Women who showed an increased plasma tryptophan ratio during bingeing ceased bingeing after the rise in tryptophan ratio occurred (Kaye et al. 1988). These women ($n = 6$) had fewer episodes of bingeing than did bulimic women ($n = 3$) who did not show an increase in plasma tryptophan.

Blood Platelet Serotonin

Weizman and colleagues (1986) reported that the density of tritium-labeled imipramine binding sites in platelets of women with anorexia nervosa ($n = 17$) was significantly lower than that in age-matched (15–18 years) control subjects ($n = 15$). Marazziti and colleagues (1988) reported that the maximum binding capacity of tritium-labeled imipramine in the platelets of bulimic women ($n = 8$) was lower than that in control subjects ($n = 7$). In a more recent study (Goldbloom et al. 1990), 23- to 25-year-old women with bulimia ($n = 22$; 8 with a history of anorexia nervosa, 3 with current depression) were compared with 20 age- and sex-matched healthy control subjects. Platelet 5-HT uptake was higher in the bulimic women than in the control subjects. If the same phenomenon occurs in the brain, there would be less 5-HT for postsynaptic receptors in the hypothalamus. No significant menstrual cycle effects were seen for either group. Only the control group showed seasonal effects in October through March and April through September, but the authors did not elaborate on the nature of these effects.

Serotonin Agonists

Studies in which tryptophan was used to treat bulimia produced inconsistent results (Krahn and Mitchell 1985; Mira and Abraham 1989). Serotonin agonist drugs, on the other hand, have been more effective than placebo in double-blind studies. The drugs used in these studies have included trazodone (Pope et al. 1989), fenfluramine (Blouin et al. 1988), and fluoxetine (Enas et al. 1989).

Summary

As Goldbloom and Garfinkel (1990) point out, many unanswered questions remain about serotonin's relationship to bulimia nervosa. As has been shown in rat studies, various serotonin agonists have different effects on eating behavior (Simansky and Vaidya 1990). "State versus trait" issues and the interaction of biological and sociocultural factors must be delineated.

Serotonin and Depression

For decades, serotonin has been implicated in the etiology of depression (Aberg-Wistedt et al. 1985; Coppen and Wood 1978), especially as it relates to the noradrenergic β-adrenergic receptor system. Intact serotonin systems are required for studies on depression and serotonin. Impaired serotonin systems prevent downregulation of β-adrenergic receptors. Serotonin systems, however, are not peculiar to depression; they are also implicated in anxious, suicidal, and impulsive states (Pies 1990). It is uncertain whether impaired serotonin systems are a primary etiological factor in depression or only a contributory factor. Furthermore, the role of serotonin systems may differ in various kinds of depression.

Plasma Tryptophan

Although plasma tryptophan levels do not seem to be decreased in depressed subjects, it is unclear whether the ratio of tryptophan to large neutral amino acids is altered. Also yet to be determined is the rate of transport and distribution of serotonin in depressed subjects compared with healthy control subjects. The literature regarding these questions has been carefully reviewed by Meltzer (1990), who reported higher plasma tryptophan levels in male depressed subjects than in female depressed subjects. Lower tryptophan levels in women would support a hypothesis for a role of serotonin in the higher incidence of depression in women than in men.

Blood Platelet Serotonin

As part of a mechanism to increase the availability of serotonin, binding sites for the neurotransmitter might be decreased. However, results of studies of tritium-labeled imipramine binding to platelet membranes and platelet serotonin uptake in depressed subjects have yielded contradictory results (Alosachie et al. 1990; Husain et al. 1991; Nemeroff et al. 1988). These studies were reviewed by Meltzer (1990). Since then, two studies have been published that reported increased platelet 5-HT2 receptors in subjects with depression (Mikuni et al. 1991; Pandey et al. 1990). The study by Pandey and colleagues (1990) also found significantly increased ^{125}I-lysergic acid diethylamide binding sites (maximal binding) in the platelets of depressed subjects with suicidal ideation or attempts ($n = 9$) compared with nonsuicidal depressed subjects ($n = 14$) and healthy control subjects ($n = 20$).

In one study, seasonal patterns of platelet serotonin uptake were found in healthy control subjects. Peak tritium-labeled imipramine binding was observed in February, and peak serotonin uptake occurred in June. Depressed subjects deviated from the normal seasonal pattern, showing lower uptake and binding (Chicz-Demet et al. 1991).

Neuroendocrine Challenge Tests

Contradictory results have been reported regarding the effects of various serotonergic agents on cortisol, prolactin, and growth hormone in depressed subjects. dl-5-Hydroxytryptophan, l-5-hydroxytryptophan, MK-212 (6-chloro-2-[1-piperazinyl]-pyrazine, a serotonin agonist), tryptophan, buspirone, and fenfluramine have been studied (Meltzer 1990; Price et al. 1991). At present, these studies lend no clarification about serotonergic mechanisms in subjects with depression. The fenfluramine study is described here in more detail for comparison with the studies on PMS and LLPDD described previously in this chapter.

Siever and colleagues (1984) studied 18 subjects with major depressive disorder according to Research Diagnostic Criteria (13 women, 5 men; mean age = 41.5 ± 2.9) and 10 age- and sex-matched control subjects (8 women, 2 men) in a double-blind, placebo-controlled study. Depressed subjects showed a significantly lower prolactin response to fenfluramine than did control subjects when prolactin response was measured as an absolute increase and as a percentage of increase from baseline prolactin levels.

Serotonin Agonists

Many serotonin uptake inhibitors have been studied for the treatment of depression. These include sertraline (Cohn et al. 1990; Koe 1990; Reimherr et al. 1990), fluoxetine (Fuller et al. 1991; Wong et al. 1990), fluvoxamine, zimeldine, paroxetine (Rickels and Schweizer 1990), clomipramine (Martensson et al. 1991), and amoxapine (Anton and Burch 1990). Serotonin agonists are effective in treating depression, but they are not more effective than other antidepressants, such as the tricyclics (Meltzer 1990).

From another perspective, perhaps most antidepressant drugs enhance 5-HT neurotransmission. In one study of 21 remitted depressed subjects receiving antidepressant therapy, 14 subjects relapsed after a tryptophan-free amino acid drink and returned to their remitted state after eating a regular diet (Delgado et al. 1990). This study suggests that serotonin may be essential for some antidepressant drug effectiveness.

Summary

Many types of evidence suggest that serotonin plays a role in the etiology of depression (Risch and Nemeroff 1992; Schatzberg and Rothschild 1992). However, it may not be the only neurotransmitter involved (Golden and Gilmore 1990).

Serotonin and Anxiety Disorders

Some data support the role of serotonin in anxiety disorders, including generalized anxiety disorder, panic disorder, and obsessive-compulsive disorder (OCD).

Neuroendocrine Challenge Tests

The indirect serotonin agonist fenfluramine was administered in one study to nine women with panic disorder, nine women with major depressive disorder, and nine control subjects who were women (Targum and Marshall 1989). In another study, fenfluramine was administered to 17 subjects with panic disorder, 12 subjects with major depressive disorder and panic disorder, 27 subjects with major depressive disorder, and 12 age- and sex-matched control subjects (Targum 1990). Women with panic disorder showed the greatest anxiogenic responses as well as greater prolactin and cortisol responses to fenfluramine. Neither study controlled for phase of the menstrual cycle.

In a study by Bastani and colleagues (1990), MK-212, 20 mg orally, and placebo were administered to 17 subjects with OCD (8 men and 9 women, ages 24–45 years) and 9 control subjects (5 men and 4 women, ages 20–55 years). Both prolactin and cortisol response were blunted in the subjects with OCD when compared with control subjects. These findings suggest diminished serotonergic responsivity in subjects with OCD.

Serotonin Agonists

A new generation of anxiolytic agents that are 5-HT$_{1A}$ receptor agonists have been developed (Eison 1989). Multiple double-blind, placebo-controlled studies have reported the superiority of buspirone over other anxiolytics for treating generalized anxiety disorder (Taylor 1990). Clomipramine is effective (Clomipramine Collaborative Study Group 1991). Fluoxetine, initiated at 5 mg daily in an open treatment study of 25 subjects with panic disorder, resulted in improvement for up to 12 months (Schneier et al. 1990). A randomized, double-blind, 8-week treatment study of 40 subjects with OCD showed that subjects given fluoxetine maleate ($n = 21$) had significantly diminished OCD symptoms than did those administered desipramine hydrochloride ($n = 19$ [Goodman et al. 1990]). Another double-blind, placebo-controlled study of 51 subjects with OCD also showed fluoxetine to be decisively helpful (Dominguez 1992).

Summary

Insel and colleagues (1990) carefully reviewed the literature regarding OCD and related serotonin not only to OCD but also to disorders of impulse control. Their rationale for the relationship between OCD and impulse control derived from their focus on phenomenology. Phenomenologically, they described subjects with OCD as inhibiting aggressive impulses because of their guilt about aggressive behaviors, in contrast to sociopaths, who do not inhibit aggressive impulses and commit crimes without experiencing guilt. These authors reasoned, then, that decreased serotonin neurotransmission is associated with a decreased capacity to suppress aggression, which results in increased expression of impulsive behaviors.

Serotonin and Other Neural Functions

Altered serotonin metabolism has been implicated in a number of other neural functions that are briefly mentioned here. In addition to those described here, a recent review article of serotonin and its possible role in schizophrenia deserves mention (Iqbal et al. 1993). (For additional details, see the references cited in this section.)

Violent Behavior

Aggressive, impulsive, and suicidal behaviors have been associated with dysfunction of the central serotonergic system (Braunig et al. 1989; Coccaro et al. 1989; Linnoila and Virkkunen 1992; Linnoila et al. 1983; Rao and Braunig 1989; Roth et al. 1990; Roy and Linnoila 1988; Traskman et al. 1981). In particular, 5-HT$_2$ receptors have been reported to be elevated in the frontal cortex of victims of violent suicide (Arora and Meltzer 1989), whereas 5-HT$_{1A}$ receptors are elevated in victims of nonviolent suicides (Meltzer 1990). These findings are consistent with results of studies reporting reduced serotonin turnover in male subjects who exhibit impulsive, aggressive behavior under the influence of alcohol (Virkkunen and Linnoila 1990) and studies implicating a biologic factor associated with an increased risk for alcoholism (Rausch et al. 1991).

Aging

In the aged brain, there is some evidence that 5-HT turnover is increased and 5-HT receptors are decreased (McEntee and Crook 1991; Roth et al. 1990). One study in animals suggested that the dysregulation that occurs with aging is presynaptic (Freo et al. 1991). Important in the assessment of changes with aging are 1) sex (Guicheney et al. 1988; McBride et al. 1990), 2) circadian rhythm of serotonin (Pietraszek et al. 1990), and 3) brain region (Gross-Isseroff et al. 1990).

Autism

Elevated platelet serotonin levels in subjects with autism have been reported by more than one group of investigators for several decades. In addition, Piven and colleagues (1991) reported that autistic subjects with siblings who had either autism or pervasive developmental disorder ($n = 5$) showed higher platelet serotonin levels than did subjects without affected siblings ($n = 23$) or healthy control subjects ($n = 10$).

Pain Perception

Serotonin regulates nociceptive input in the periphery through 5-HT$_3$ receptors by depolarizing afferent fibers, thereby causing pain (Humphrey et al. 1990; Richardson 1990). Conversely, it inhibits pain transmission and increases pain gating in the spinal cord through 5-HT$_1$–like receptors and in the brain stem through 5-HT$_2$ receptors (Richardson 1990). In a study by Shanks and colleagues (1991), pain-provoked changes in serotonin levels in the brains of six mouse strains were most evident in the mesocortex.

Temperature Regulation

Early reports in animals documented pyrogenic effects of serotonin (Horita and Gogerty 1958). In a later study (Huang et al.
1990), serotonin was said to induce hypothermia. However,
when serotonin neurons of the dorsal raphe nuclei in cats were
examined after increased ambient temperature and pyrogen-
induced fever, no changes in the activity of brain serotonergic
neurons were noted (Jacobs et al. 1990). It is currently believed
that the 5-HT$_{1A}$ receptor is associated with hypothermia in humans (Lesch et al. 1990) and that the 5-HT$_2$ receptor is associated with hyperthermia in rodents.

Sleep Regulation

Serotonin plays a role in regulating sleep (Morgane and Stern
1978), probably acting as a neurotransmitter to suppress
wakefulness and to antagonize the arousal effects of catechola-
mines (Wauquier and Dugovic 1990). In addition, serotonin
may act as a neurohormone to liberate hypnogenic factors (Wauquier and Dugovic 1990). In one study, however, nighttime administration of *m*-chlorophenylpiperazine, a serotonin agonist,
reduced total sleep time and sleep efficiency in all six healthy
volunteers studied (Lawlor et al. 1991). In that study, slow-wave
sleep and rapid eye movement sleep were decreased and Stage I
sleep was prolonged in most of the subjects.

Sexual Behavior

In rats, serotonin can both inhibit and facilitate sexual behavior,
depending on which receptor subtypes are activated. The 5-HT$_2$
receptors are thought to be predominantly inhibitory (Gorzalka
et al. 1990). In humans, the role of serotonin in sexual behavior
is less clear. Anecdotal reports of orgasm dysfunction, however,
have been reported in subjects being treated with serotonergic
agents (Zajeck et al. 1991).

 One retrospective study of 13 subjects who sought treatment
for sexual symptoms and were treated with serotonin reuptake

blockers has been published. Subjects with paraphilia showed moderate improvement with treatment (Stein et al. 1992).

Immunological Responsivity

Serotonin is thought to participate in the regulation of immunity. Rats with high platelet serotonin contents showed better immune reactions to sheep erythrocytes than did rats with low platelet serotonin contents (Poljak-Blazi et al. 1990). In humans, the specific binding to lymphocytes of tritium-labeled serotonin was significantly lower in subjects with Alzheimer's disease than in age-matched control subjects without dementia and was lower in children with idiopathic mental retardation than in healthy children (Singh et al. 1990).

Conclusions

Alterations of serotonin regulation seem to be correlated with particular psychopathological behaviors or symptoms, rather than with particular diagnostic disorders (van Praag et al. 1987). They are correlated with depressed mood, increased anxiety, aggressive behaviors, and changes in eating and sleep behaviors and pain perception, which are found in a number of psychiatric disorders (depression, LLPDD, bulimia nervosa, anxiety disorders, alcoholism). The symptoms produced by diminished serotonin levels can best be conceptualized as secondary to decreased inhibitory control, rather than as secondary to altered activatory control (Soubrie 1986). The serotonergic system, then, might be conceptualized as modulating various target structures in the body (e.g., pain perception, temperature regulation, sleep regulation) in conjunction with the person's level of arousal (Jacobs et al. 1990).

Because alterations in serotonin regulation have been correlated with particular behaviors and symptoms of LLPDD, it is tempting to hypothesize that the serotonergic system has some relationship to the etiology of LLPDD. This speculation is described more fully in Chapter 11. Proof of such a hypothesis will rest on studies demonstrating actual brain differences, both metabolic and anatomic, between women with and women without LLPDD.

References

Aberg-Wistedt A, Wistedt B, Bertilsson L: Higher CSF levels of HVA and 5-HIAA in delusional compared to nondelusional depression. Arch Gen Psychiatry 42:925–926, 1985

Alosachie I, Peter JB, Tsuchihashi H, et al: Decreased imipramine binding by platelet membranes in major depression is not associated with plasma autoantibodies to imipramine binding sites. Biol Psychiatry 28:365–368, 1990

Anton RF Jr, Burch EA Jr: A comparison of amoxapine versus amitriptyline plus perphenazine in the treatment of psychotic depression. Am J Psychiatry 147:1203–1208, 1990

Arora RC, Meltzer HY: Serotonergic measures in suicide brain, III: increased 5-HT$_2$ binding sites in frontal cortex of suicide victims. Am J Psychiatry 146:730–736, 1989

Ashby CR Jr, Carr LA, Cook CL, et al: Alteration of platelet serotonergic mechanism and monoamine oxidase activity in premenstrual syndrome. Biol Psychiatry 24:225–233, 1988

Ashby CR Jr, Carr LA, Cook CL, et al: Alteration of 5-HT uptake by plasma fractions in the premenstrual syndrome. J Neural Transm Gen Sect 79:41–50, 1990

Ashby CR Jr, Carr LA, Cook CL, et al: Inhibition of serotonin uptake in rat brain synaptosomes by plasma from patients with premenstrual syndrome. Biol Psychiatry 31:1169–1171, 1992

Awouters F, Niemegeers CJE, Megens AAHP, et al: Functional interaction between serotonin-S$_2$ and dopamine-D$_2$ neurotransmission as revealed by selective antagonism of hyper-reactivity to tryptamine and apomorphine. J Pharmacol Exp Ther 254:945–951, 1990

Bancroft J, Cook A, Davidson D, et al: Blunting of neuroendocrine responses to infusion of L-tryptophan in women with perimenstrual mood change. Psychol Med 21:305–312, 1991

Bastani B, Nash F, Meltzer HY: Prolactin and cortisol responses to MK-212, a serotonin agonist, in obsessive-compulsive disorder. Arch Gen Psychiatry 47:833–839, 1990

Belmaker RH, Murphy DL, Wyatt RJ, et al: Human platelet monoamine oxidase changes during the menstrual cycle. Arch Gen Psychiatry 31:553–556, 1974

Blouin AG, Blouin JH, Perez EL, et al: Treatment of bulimia with fenfluramine and desipramine. J Clin Psychopharmacol 8:261–269, 1988

Braunig P, Rao ML, Fimmers R: Blood serotonin levels in suicidal schizophrenic patients. Acta Psychiatr Scand 79:186–189, 1989

Briggs M, Briggs M: Relationship between monoamine oxidase activity and sex hormone concentration in human blood plasma. J Reprod Fertil 29:447–450, 1972

Brzezinski AA, Wurtman JJ, Wurtman RJ, et al: d-Fenfluramine suppresses the increased calorie and carbohydrate intakes and improves the mood of women with premenstrual depression. Obstet Gynecol 76:296–301, 1990

Chicz-Demet A, Reist C, Demet EM: Relationship between seasonal patterns of platelet serotonin uptake and ^{3}H-imipramine binding in depressed patients and normal controls. Prog Neuropsychopharmacol Biol Psychiatry 15:25–39, 1991

Clomipramine Collaborative Study Group: Clomipramine in the treatment of patients with obsessive-compulsive disorder. Arch Gen Psychiatry 48:730–738, 1991

Coccaro EF, Siever LJ, Klar HM, et al: Serotonergic studies in patients with affective and personality disorders. Arch Gen Psychiatry 46:587–599, 1989

Coccaro EF, Gabriel S, Mahon T, et al: Preliminary evidence of a serotonin (5-HT-1–like) component to the prolactin response to buspirone challenge in humans. Arch Gen Psychiatry 47:594–595, 1990

Cohn CK, Shrivastava R, Mendels J, et al: Double-blind, multicenter comparison of sertraline and amitriptyline in elderly depressed patients. J Clin Psychiatry 51 (suppl B):28–33, 1990

Colwell CS: Light and serotonin interact in affecting the circadian system of Aplysia. J Comp Physiol [A] 167:841–845, 1990

Coppen A, Wood K: Tryptophan and depressive illness. Psychol Med 8:49–57, 1978

David D, Freeman A, Harrington TM, et al: Buspirone for anxious women in a primary care environment: a multicenter open evaluation. Advances in Therapy 4:251–264, 1987

Delgado PL, Charney DS, Price LH, et al: Serotonin function and the mechanism of antidepressant action. Arch Gen Psychiatry 47:411–418, 1990

de Tejada AL, Carreno E, Lopez L, et al: Eliminacion urinaria de acido 5-hidroxi-indol acetico durante el ciclo menstrual humano. Ginecol Obstet Mex 44:85–91, 1978

Dominguez RA: Serotonergic antidepressants and their efficacy in obsessive compulsive disorder. J Clin Psychiatry 53 (suppl):56–59, 1992

Eison MS: The new generation of serotonin anxiolytic agents: possible clinical roles. Psychopathology 22 (suppl 1):13–20, 1989

Ellis PM, McIntosh CJ, Cooke RR: Variation of platelet [^{3}H]imipramine binding during the menstrual cycle in healthy young women. Human Psychopharmacology 7:51–54, 1992

Enas GG, Pope HG, Levine LR: Fluoxetine in bulimia nervosa: double blind study. Paper presented at the 142nd annual meeting of the American Psychiatric Association, San Francisco, CA, May 1989

Engel GL: The clinical application of the biopsychosocial model. Am J Psychiatry 137:535–544, 1980

Eriksson E, Sundblad C, Lisjo P, et al: Premenstrual syndrome: (1) enhanced plasma levels of free testosterone, (2) symptom reduction by means of a serotonin reuptake inhibitor. Neuroendocrinology Letters 12:284, 1990

Feine R, Belmaker RH, Rimon R, et al: Platelet monoamine oxidase in women with premenstrual syndrome. Neuropsychobiology 3:105–110, 1977

Fischette CT, Biegon A, McEwen BS: Sex steroid modulation of the serotonin behavioral syndrome. Life Sci 35:1197–1206, 1984

Freo U, Rapoport SI, Soncrant TT: Age-related alterations in behavioral and cerebral metabolic responses to the serotonin agonist meta-chlorophenylpiperazine in rats. Neurobiol Aging 12:137–144, 1991

Fuller RW, Wong DT, Robertson DW: Fluoxetine: a selective inhibitor of serotonin uptake. Med Res Rev 11:17–34, 1991

Gilman AG, Goodman LS, Rall TW, et al: The Pharmacological Basis of Therapeutics. New York, Macmillan, 1985

Gingras JL, Lawson EE, McNamara MC: Developmental characteristics in the daily rhythm of serotonin concentration within rabbit brainstem regions. Dev Pharmacol Ther 14:245–253, 1990

Glennon RA, Darmani NA, Martin BR: Multiple populations of serotonin receptors may modulate the behavioral effects of serotonergic agents. Life Sci 48:2493–2498, 1991

Goldbloom DS, Garfinkel PE: The serotonin hypothesis of bulimia nervosa: theory and evidence. Can J Psychiatry 35:741–744, 1990

Goldbloom DS, Hicks LK, Garfinkel PE: Platelet serotonin uptake in bulimia nervosa. Biol Psychiatry 28:644–647, 1990

Golden RN, Gilmore JH: Serotonin and mood disorders. Psychiatric Annals 20:580–586, 1990

Goodman WK, Price LH, Delgado PL, et al: Specificity of serotonin reuptake inhibitors in the treatment of obsessive-compulsive disorder. Arch Gen Psychiatry 47:577–585, 1990

Goodwin GM, Fairburn CG, Cowen PJ: Dieting changes serotonergic function in women, not men: implications for the etiology of anorexia nervosa? Psychol Med 17:839–842, 1987

Gorzalka BB, Mendelson SD, Watson NV: Serotonin receptor subtypes and sexual behavior. Ann N Y Acad Sci 600:435–479, 1990

Gross-Isseroff R, Salama D, Israeli M, et al: Autoradiographic analysis of age-dependent changes in serotonin 5-HT$_2$ receptors of the human brain postmortem. Brain Res 519:223–227, 1990

Guicheney P, Leger D, Barrat J, et al: Platelet serotonin content and plasma tryptophan in peri- and postmenopausal women: variations with plasma oestrogen levels and depressive symptoms. Eur J Clin Invest 18:297–304, 1988

Halbreich U, Rojansky N, Wang K: Psychological, hormonal and neurotransmitter aspects of menstrually related symptoms, in Headache and Depression: Serotonin Pathways as a Common Clue. Edited by Nappi G, Bono G, Sandrini G, et al. New York, Raven, 1991, pp 191–203

Hallman J, Oreland L, Edman G, et al: Thrombocyte monoamine oxidase activity and personality traits in women with severe premenstrual syndrome. Acta Psychiatr Scand 76:225–234, 1987

Harrison WM, Endicott J, Rabkin JG, et al: Treatment of premenstrual dysphoric changes: clinical outcome and methodological implications. Psychopharmacol Bull 20:118–122, 1984

Horita A, Gogerty JH: The pyretogenic effect of 5-hydroxytryptophan and its comparison with that of LSD. J Pharmacol Exp Ther 122:195–200, 1958

Huang Q, Matsuda H, Sakai K, et al: The effect of ginger on serotonin induced hypothermia and diarrhea. Yakugaku Zasshi 110:936–942, 1990

Huff BB, Dowd AL (eds): Physicians' Desk Reference. Oradell, NJ, Medical Economics, 1988

Humphrey PPA, Feniuk W, Perren MJ, et al: Serotonin and migraine. Ann N Y Acad Sci 600:587–600, 1990

Husain MM, Knight DL, Doraiswamy PM, et al: Platelet [^{3}H]-imipramine binding and leukoencephalopathy in geriatric depression. Biol Psychiatry 29:665–670, 1991

Insel TR, Zohar J, Benkelfat C, et al: Serotonin in obsessions, compulsions, and the control of aggressive impulses. Ann N Y Acad Sci 600:574–586, 1990

Iqbal N, Goldsamt LA, Wetzler S, et al: Serotonin and schizophrenia. Psychiatric Annals 23:186–192, 1993

Jacobs BL, Wilkinson LO, Fornal CA: The role of brain serotonin. Neuropsychopharmacology 3:473–479, 1990

Jimerson DC, Lesem MD, Hegg AP, et al: Serotonin in human eating disorders. Ann N Y Acad Sci 600:532–544, 1990

Kaye WH, Gwirtsman HE, Brewerton TD, et al: Binging behavior and plasma amino acids: a possible involvement of brain serotonin in bulimia nervosa. Psychiatry Res 23:31–43, 1988

Klaiber EL, Kobayashi Y, Broverman DM, et al: Plasma monoamine oxidase activity in regularly menstruating women and in amenorrheic women receiving cyclic treatment with estrogens and a progestin. J Clin Endocrinol Metab 33:630–638, 1971

Koe BK: Preclinical pharmacology of sertraline: a potent and specific inhibitor of serotonin reuptake. J Clin Psychiatry 51 (suppl B):13–17, 1990

Krahn D, Mitchell J: Use of L-tryptophan in treating bulimia. Am J Psychiatry 142:1130, 1985

Labrum AH: Hypothalamic, pineal and pituitary factors in the premenstrual syndrome. J Reprod Med 28:438–445, 1983

Lawlor BA, Newhouse PA, Balkin TJ, et al: A preliminary study of the effects of nighttime administration of the serotonin agonist, m-CPP, on sleep architecture and behavior in healthy volunteers. Biol Psychiatry 29:281–286, 1991

Lepage P, Steiner M: Gender and serotonergic dysregulation: implications for late luteal phase dysphoric disorder, in Serotonin-Related Psychiatric Syndromes: Clinical and Therapeutic Links. Edited by Cassano GB, Akiskal HS. London, Royal Society of Medicine, 1991, pp 1271–1277

Lesch KP, Mayer S, Disselkamp-Tietze J, et al: Subsensitivity of the 5-hydroxytryptamine$_{1A}$ (5-HT$_{1A}$) receptor-mediated hypothermic response to ipsapirone in unipolar depression. Life Sci 46:1271–1277, 1990

Linnoila VMI, Virkkunen M: Aggression, suicidality, and serotonin. J Clin Psychiatry 53 (suppl):46–51, 1992

Linnoila M, Virkkunen M, Scheinin M, et al: Low cerebrospinal fluid 5-hydroxyindoleacetic acid concentration differentiates impulsive from nonimpulsive violent behavior. Life Sci 33:2609–2614, 1983

Lydiard RB, Brady KT, O'Neil PM, et al: Precursor amino acid concentrations in normal weight bulimics and normal controls. Prog Neuropsychopharmacol Biol Psychiatry 12:893–898, 1988

Marazziti D, Macchi E, Rotondo A, et al: Involvement of serotonin system in bulimia. Life Sci 43:2123–2126, 1988

Marazziti D, Falcone MF, Castrogiovanni P, et al: Seasonal serotonin uptake changes in healthy subjects. Mol Chem Neuropathol 13:145–153, 1990

Martensson B, Wagner A, Beck O, et al: Effects of clomipramine treatment on cerebrospinal fluid monoamine metabolites and platelet ^{3}H-imipramine binding and serotonin uptake concentration in major depressive disorder. Acta Psychiatr Scand 83:123–133, 1991

McBride PA, Tierney H, DeMeo M, et al: Effects of age and gender on CNS serotonergic responsivity in normal adults. Biol Psychiatry 27:1143–1155, 1990

McEntee WJ, Crook TH: Serotonin, memory, and the aging brain. Psychopharmacology 103:143–149, 1991

McEwen BS, Parsons B: Gonadal steroid action on the brain: neurochemistry and neuropharmacology. Annu Rev Pharmacol Toxicol 22:555–598, 1982

McGuire M: The chemistry of charisma. Science Digest 91:77, 1983

Meltzer HY: Role of serotonin in depression. Ann N Y Acad Sci 600:486–499, 1990

Menkes DB, Taghavi E, Mason PA, et al: Fluoxetine treatment of severe premenstrual syndrome. Br Med J 305:346–347, 1992

Mikuni M, Kusumi I, Kagaya A, et al: Increased 5-HT-2 receptor function as measured by serotonin stimulated phosphoinositide hydrolysis in platelets of depressed patients. Prog Neuropsychopharmacol Biol Psychiatry 15:49–61, 1991

Mira M, Abraham S: L-tryptophan as an adjunct to treatment of bulimia nervosa. Lancet 2:1162–1163, 1989

Moline ML, Severino SK, Wagner DR, et al: Response to fenfluramine in premenstrual syndrome, in New Research Program and Abstracts: American Psychiatric Association 145th Annual Meeting, Washington, DC, May 1992, Abstract #535, p 178

Moore RY: The circadian timing system and the organization of sleep-wake behavior, in Handbook of Sleep Disorders. Edited by Thorpy MJ. New York, Marcel Dekker, 1990, pp 103–115

Morgane PJ, Stern WC: Serotonin in the regulation of sleep, in Serotonin in Health and Disease, II: Physiological Regulation and Pharmacological Action. Edited by Essman W. New York, Spectrum, 1978, pp 205–245

Morin LP, Michels KM, Smale L, et al: Serotonin regulation of circadian rhythmicity. Ann N Y Acad Sci 600:418–426, 1990

Nemeroff CB, Knight DL, Krishnan KRR, et al: Marked reduction in the number of platelet [^{3}H]-imipramine binding sites in geriatric depression. Arch Gen Psychiatry 45:919–923, 1988

Odink J, Van der Ploeg HM, Van den Berg H, et al: Circadian and circatrigintan rhythms of biogenic amines in premenstrual syndrome (PMS). Psychosom Med 52:346–356, 1990

Pandey GN, Pandey SC, Janicak PG, et al: Platelet serotonin-2 receptor binding sites in depression and suicide. Biol Psychiatry 28:215–222, 1990

Pies R: Serotonin: the neurotransmitter of the 1990s. Psychiatric Times, October 1990, pp 30–32

Pietraszek MH, Urano T, Serizawa K, et al: Circadian rhythm of serotonin: influence of age. Thromb Res 60:253–257, 1990

Piven J, Tsai G, Nehme E, et al: Platelet serotonin, a possible marker for familial autism. J Autism Dev Disord 21:51–59, 1991

Poljak-Blazi M, Jernej B, Cicin-Sain L, et al: Immunological response of rats selected for high or low platelet serotonin content. Periodicum Biologorum 92:189–190, 1990

Pope HG, Keck PE, McElroy SI, et al: A placebo-controlled study of trazodone in bulimia nervosa. J Clin Psychopharmacol 9:254–259, 1989

Price WA, Giannini AJ, Seng CS: Use of L-tryptophan in the treatment of premenstrual tension: a case report. Psychiatric Forum 13:44–46, 1984–1985

Price LH, Charney DS, Delgado PL, et al: Serotonin function and depression: neuroendocrine and mood responses to intravenous L-tryptophan in depressed patients and healthy comparison subjects. Am J Psychiatry 148:1518–1525, 1991

Prosser RA, Miller JD, Heller HC: A serotonin agonist phase-shifts the circadian clock in the suprachiasmatic nuclei in vitro. Brain Res 534:336–339, 1990

Rao ML, Braunig P: Peripheral serotonin and catecholamine levels and suicidal behavior, in New Directions in Affective Disorders. Edited by Lerer B, Gershon S. New York, Springer, 1989, pp 320–325

Rao ML, Muller-Oerlinghausen B, Mackert A, et al: The influence of phototherapy on serotonin and melatonin in non-seasonal depression. Pharmacopsychiatry 23:155–158, 1990

Rapkin AJ, Edelmuth E, Chang LC, et al: Whole-blood serotonin in premenstrual syndrome. Obstet Gynecol 70:533–537, 1987

Rapkin AJ, Buckman TD, Stuphin MS, et al: Platelet monoamine oxidase B activity in women with premenstrual syndrome. Am J Obstet Gynecol 159:1536–1540, 1988

Rausch JL, Monteiro MG, Schuckit MA: Platelet serotonin uptake in men with family histories of alcoholism. Neuropsychopharmacology 4:83–86, 1991

Reimherr FW, Chouinard G, Cohn CK, et al: Antidepressant efficacy of sertraline: a double-blind, placebo and amitriptyline-controlled, multicenter comparison study in outpatients with major depression. J Clin Psychiatry 51:18–27, 1990

Richardson BP: Serotonin and nociception. Ann N Y Acad Sci 600:511–520, 1990

Rickels K, Schweizer E: Clinical overview of serotonin reuptake inhibitors. J Clin Psychiatry 51 (suppl B):9–12, 1990

Rickels K, Freeman E, Sondheimer S: Buspirone in treatment of premenstrual syndrome. Lancet 1:777, 1989

Rickels K, Freeman EW, Sondheimer S, et al: Fluoxetine in the treatment of premenstrual syndrome. Current Therapeutic Research 48:161–166, 1990

Risch SC, Nemeroff CB: Neurochemical alterations of serotonergic neuronal systems in depression. J Clin Psychiatry 53 (suppl):3–7, 1992

Rojansky N, Halbreich U, Zander K, et al: Imipramine receptor binding and serotonin uptake in platelets of women with premenstrual changes. Gynecol Obstet Invest 31:146–152, 1991

Roth BL, Hamblin M, Ciaranello RD: Regulation of 5-HT$_2$ and 5-HT$_{1C}$ serotonin receptor levels. Neuropsychopharmacology 3:427–433, 1990

Roy A, Linnoila M: Suicidal behavior, impulsiveness and serotonin. Acta Psychiatr Scand 78:529–535, 1988

Schatzberg AF, Rothschild AJ: Serotonin activity in psychotic (delusional) major depression. J Clin Psychiatry 53 (suppl):52–55, 1992

Schneier FR, Liebowitz MR, Davies SO, et al: Fluoxetine in panic disorder. J Clin Psychopharmacol 10:119–121, 1990

Schreiber W, Schweiger U, Werner D, et al: Circadian pattern of large neutral amino acids, glucose, insulin, and food intake in anorexia nervosa and bulimia nervosa. Metabolism 40:503–507, 1991

Shanks N, Zalcman S, Zacharko RM, et al: Alterations of central norepinephrine, dopamine and serotonin in several strains of mice following acute stressor exposure. Pharmacol Biochem Behav 38:69–75, 1991

Siever LJ, Murphy DL, Slater S, et al: Plasma prolactin changes following fenfluramine in depressed patients compared to controls: an evaluation of central serotonergic responsivity in depression. Life Sci 34:1029–1039, 1984

Simansky KJ, Vaidya AH: Behavioral mechanisms for the anorectic action of the serotonin (5-HT) uptake inhibitor sertraline in rats: comparison with directly acting 5-HT agonists. Brain Res Bull 25:953–960, 1990

Singh VK, Warren RP, Singh EA: Binding of [^{3}H] serotonin to lymphocytes in patients with neuropsychiatric disorders. Mol Chem Neuropathol 13:167–173, 1990

Soubrie P: Reconciling the role of central serotonin neurons in human and animal behavior. Behavioral Brain Science 9:319–364, 1986

Stahl SM, Ciaranello RD, Berger PA: Platelet serotonin in schizophrenia and depression, in Advances in Biochemical Psychopharmacology, Vol 34. Edited by Ho BT, Schoolar JC, Usdin E. New York, Raven, 1982, pp 183–198

Steege JF, Stout AL, Knight DL, et al: Reduced platelet tritium-labeled imipramine binding sites in women with premenstrual syndrome. Am J Obstet Gynecol 167:168–172, 1992

Stein DJ, Hollander E, Anthony DT, et al: Serotonergic medications for sexual obsessions, sexual addictions, and paraphilia. J Clin Psychiatry 53:267–271, 1992

Stone AB, Pearlstein TB, Brown WA: Fluoxetine in the treatment of late luteal phase dysphoric disorder. J Clin Psychiatry 52:290–293, 1991

Sundblad C, Modigh K, Andersch B, et al: Clomipramine effectively reduces premenstrual irritability and dysphoria—a placebo-controlled trial. Acta Psychiatr Scand 85:39–47, 1992

Tam WYK, Chan M-Y, Lee PHK: The menstrual cycle and platelet 5-HT uptake. Psychosom Med 47:352–362, 1985

Targum SD: Differential responses to anxiogenic challenge studies in patients with major depressive disorder and panic disorder. Biol Psychiatry 28:21–34, 1990

Targum SD, Marshall LE: Fenfluramine provocation of anxiety in patients with panic disorder. Psychiatr Res 28:295–306, 1989

Taylor DP: Serotonin agents in anxiety. Ann N Y Acad Sci 600:545–557, 1990

Taylor DL, Mathew RJ, Ho BT, et al: Serotonin levels and platelet uptake during premenstrual tension. Neuropsychobiology 12:16–18, 1984

Traskman L, Esberg M, Bertilsson L, et al: Monoamine metabolites in CSF and suicidal behavior. Arch Gen Psychiatry 38:631–636, 1981

van Praag HM, Kahn RS, Asnis GM, et al: Denosologization of biological psychiatry or the specificity of 5-HT disturbances in psychiatric disorders. J Affect Disord 13:1–8, 1987

Veeninga AT, Westenberg HGM: Serotonergic function and late luteal phase dysphoric disorder. Psychopharmacology 108:153–158, 1992

Veeninga AT, Westenberg HGM, Weusten JTN: Fluvoxamine in the treatment of menstrually related mood disorders. Psychopharmacology 102:414–416, 1990

Virkkunen M, Linnoila M: Serotonin in early onset, male alcoholics with violent behaviour. Ann Med 22:327–331, 1990

Wauquier A, Dugovic C: Serotonin and sleep-wakefulness. Ann N Y Acad Sci 600:447–459, 1990

Weizman R, Carmi M, Tyano S, et al: High affinity [^{3}H] imipramine binding and serotonin uptake to platelets of adolescent females suffering from anorexia nervosa. Life Sci 38:1235–1242, 1986

Wong DT, Fuller RW, Robertson DW: Fluoxetine and its two enantiomers as selective serotonin uptake inhibitors. Acta Pharm Nord 2:171–180, 1990

Wood SH, Mortola JF, Chan Y-F, et al: Treatment of premenstrual syndrome with fluoxetine: a double-blind, placebo-controlled, crossover study. Obstet Gynecol 80:339–344, 1992

Wurtman J: Serotonin agonist may ease some PMS symptoms. Clinical Psychiatry News, June 1990, p 16

Yatham LN, Barry S, Dinan TG: Serotonin receptors, buspirone, and premenstrual syndrome. Lancet 2:1447–1448, 1989

Zajeck J, Fawcett J, Schaff M, et al: The role of serotonin in sexual dysfunction: fluoxetine-associated orgasm dysfunction. J Clin Psychiatry 52:66–68, 1991

ℑ 5 ℜ

Treatment Efficacy

Ana Rivera-Tovar, Ph.D., Renee Rhodes, B.A.,
Teri B. Pearlstein, M.D., and Ellen Frank, Ph.D.

> The whole area of bio versus psycho versus social will
> probably remain central to psychiatry for a while, and an
> area where we are at risk of major premature closures.
> One could call the risk intellectual and clinical segrega-
> tion rather than integration.
>
> Can we cooperate? It is easy to denigrate those who
> think differently, or who know different things.
>
> Hartmann 1992, p. 1139

Approaches to treating premenstrual mood and physical disturbances date back more than 60 years, when Frank (1931)
first coined the term "premenstrual tension." This review of
treatment studies focuses on those research studies in which specific diagnostic criteria were used to screen subjects and confirm
a diagnosis of premenstrual syndrome (PMS)/late luteal phase
dysphoric disorder (LLPDD), and/or those in which adequate
control conditions were compared with active treatment. Generally, treatment strategies mirror the numerous proposed etiolo-

This work was supported in part by Grant 5-30915 from the National Institute of
Mental Health Clinical Research Center and Grant 5-36460 from the John D. and
Catherine T. MacArthur Foundation.

gies of PMS/LLPDD. In this chapter, we divide these varied approaches into somatic and psychosocial treatments.

Somatic Treatments

Most of the somatic treatment studies reviewed here have been selected on the basis of their use of DSM-III-R (American Psychiatric Association 1987) diagnostic criteria for LLPDD. In other cases, the following criteria have been used: at least 1 month of pretreatment prospective symptom ratings to verify the diagnosis of PMS; studies designed in a double-blind, crossover manner, so that subjects essentially act as their own control subjects; and studies that suggest a specific etiology, enlisting subjects known to be nonresponsive to placebo treatment. The studies of somatic treatments are grouped into the following seven categories:

1. Ovulation suppressants
2. Progesterone and dydrogesterone
3. Nutritional supplements
4. Diuretics
5. Psychopharmacologic agents
6. Melatonin inhibitors
7. Miscellaneous treatments

Ovulation Suppressants

Many treatments effectively reduce or eliminate the symptoms of PMS by suppressing ovulation. Table 5–1 lists these treatments, such as danazol, luteinizing hormone–releasing hormone agonists, estradiol plus norethisterone, and oophorectomy.

Danazol is a gonadotropin-releasing hormone agonist that probably exerts its effects by suppressing the gonadotropin surge at ovulation (Watts et al. 1987). Of the four studies reviewed here, two were designed in a double-blind, crossover manner. In the first, Gilmore and colleagues (1985) found that danazol (400 mg daily) was superior to placebo, but side effects were a problem for many

Table 5–1. Ovulation suppression

Reference	Treatment	Measures	Methods	Results
Gilmore et al. 1985	Danazol	MDQ	36 women; 400 mg danazol or placebo daily for 3 mo; MDQ daily	Danazol superior to placebo
Sarno et al. 1987	Danazol	MSD	14 women; 200 mg danazol or placebo daily, from onset of symptoms until menses, for 2 mo	Danazol superior to placebo
Watts et al. 1985	Danazol	Total wk 4 score of each symptom; cyclical change scores (wk 4/wk 2)	100 ($n = 10$), 200 ($n = 10$), or 400 ($n = 10$) mg danazol or placebo ($n = 10$) daily for 3 mo	Danazol superior to placebo on 5 of the 7 symptoms studied
Watts et al. 1987	Danazol	Total wk 4 score of each symptom; cyclical change scores (wk 4/wk 2)	100 ($n = 10$), 200 ($n = 10$), or 400 ($n = 10$) mg danazol or placebo ($n = 10$) daily for 3 mo	200- and 400-mg doses best for cyclical irritability; 400-mg dose best for weekly irritability; breast pain lower on all danazol doses
Muse et al. 1984	LHRH agonist	Premenstrual assessment calendar; plasma LH, FSH, estradiol, and progesterone	8 women; 50 µg LHRH agonist or placebo daily for 3 mo	Active treatment superior to placebo for reducing only physical symptoms and abolishing cyclical hormone fluctuations
Bancroft et al. 1987	LHRH agonist (buserelin)	VAS; urinary estrogen and pregnanediol	600 µg nasal buserelin daily for 18–65 wks ($n = 10$) or 3–11 wks ($n = 10$); 5 long-term placebo once symptoms were under control	No change in hormones; improvement in mood, bloating, and breast tenderness for long-term treatment; no differences for short-term treatment
Hammarbäck and Bäckström 1988	LHRH agonist (buserelin)	Plasma estrogen and progesterone; VAS	23 women; 400 µg nasal buserelin or placebo daily for 3 mo; blood samples weekly	No changes in hormones; buserelin superior to placebo for all symptoms

(continued)

Table 5–1. Ovulation suppression *(continued)*

Reference	Treatment	Measures	Methods	Results
Magos et al. 1986	Estradiol + norethisterone	MDQ; retrospective VAS; General Health Questionnaire	68 women; 100 mg estradiol sc + 5 mg norethisterone po for 7 days, 9 days before menses; physician review every 3 mo; MDQs daily	Based on MDQ, active Tx superior to placebo; no differences on any other measures
Watson et al. 1989	Estradiol + norethisterone	MDQ; PDQ	40 women; 200 µg estradiol sc + 5 mg norethisterone or placebo for 3 mo; questionnaires daily	Active treatment superior to placebo
Casper and Hearn 1990	Oophorectomy and hysterectomy + estrogen	PRISM; Campbell's Overall Life Satisfaction (Campbell et al. 1976); Index of General Affect (Campbell et al. 1976); POMS; Quality of Life Questionnaire (Evans et al. 1985)	14 women with treatment-resistant PMS; oophorectomy and hysterectomy performed on all women but one, who had already had hysterectomy; 6-week follow-up and PRISM calendar completed at 6 mo	Surgical intervention eliminated premenstrual symptoms
Casson et al. 1990	Oophorectomy and hysterectomy + estrogen	PRISM	14 women with treatment-resistant PMS; oophorectomy and hysterectomy performed; PRISM calendar completed at two points during a follow-up year	Surgical intervention eliminated premenstrual symptoms

Note.   FSH = follicle-stimulating hormone. LH = luteinizing hormone. LHRH = luteinizing hormone–releasing hormone. MDQ = Menstrual Distress Questionnaire (Moos 1968). MSQ = Menstrual Symptom Questionnaire (Abraham 1980). PDQ = Personality Diagnostic Questionnaire (Magos et al. 1986). POMS = Profile of Mood States (McNair et al. 1971). PRISM = Prospective Record of the Impact and Severity of Menstrual Symptomatology (Reid 1985). VAS = visual analog scale.

of the 36 women completing the study. Sarno and colleagues (1987) studied a lower dose of danazol (200 mg daily), which was given only in the presence of premenstrual symptoms. This lower, cyclical dose of danazol was also superior to placebo for symptom relief, but without the side effects noted in the study by Gilmore and colleagues (1985). The Sarno team's study raises the question of what is the mechanism of action of danazol, because treatment during the luteal phase would not block ovulation. In two single-blind, randomized studies, Watts and colleagues (1985, 1987) looked at the efficacy of danazol in subjects receiving doses of 100, 200, and 400 mg compared with a control group receiving placebo. Once again, danazol was superior to placebo, with side effects becoming problematic at the high dose.

The results of these four studies suggest that a relatively low, cyclical dose of danazol has effects comparable to those of high doses but is better tolerated. In addition, cyclical administration of danazol seems to maintain estradiol and gonadotropin at normal levels throughout the menstrual cycle.

Table 5–1 summarizes the results of two studies of estradiol plus norethisterone. One study, by Watson and colleagues (1989), was performed in a double-blind, crossover manner, using implants of placebo or 200 mg of estradiol. Magos and colleagues (1986) used a 100-mg estradiol implant or placebo in a double-blind, longitudinal study. In both studies, daily scores from the Menstrual Distress Questionnaire (Moos 1968) provided a measure of treatment outcome. Also common to both studies was the use of oral norethisterone (5 mg daily), taken by subjects premenstrually to promote normal menstruation. In both studies, estradiol plus norethisterone was superior to placebo for relief of premenstrual symptoms. Watson and colleagues (1989) found that some women experienced skin irritation and discoloration at the site of the estradiol patch. Although Magos and colleagues (1986) noted no side effects with the estradiol implants, they warned of the possibility of hyperestrogenemia with this form of treatment.

The efficacy of buserelin, a luteinizing hormone–releasing hormone agonist, was tested in three studies, with mixed results. Hammarbäck and Bäckström (1988) performed the only double-blind crossover trial, in which buserelin (400 μg daily) or placebo was administered by nasal spray and symptoms were rated daily on a visual analog scale. These authors found buserelin to be superior to placebo for all symptoms studied. At the 400-μg daily dose, women became anovulatory while continuing to menstruate regularly, with no development of postmenopausal symptoms. Bancroft and colleagues (1987) also used nasal-spray administration in their placebo-controlled trial of buserelin (600 μg daily). Active treatment was given for long-term ($n = 10$) and short-term ($n = 10$) periods. Five women from the long-term group received placebo after their symptoms had stabilized while receiving buserelin. The results of this study were mixed, with buserelin superior for mood symptoms, bloating, and breast tenderness, but not for irritability and low energy. In addition, many side effects, including hot flushes, labile mood, hypomania, and loss of libido, were seen in the subjects. Muse and colleagues (1984) used a daily injection of 50 μg of a luteinizing hormone–releasing hormone agonist or placebo in a single-blind, crossover study, in which the efficacy of buserelin was demonstrated only for physical symptoms. Hot flushes were a side effect of treatment in this study, and the authors also cautioned that osteoporosis may develop if this treatment is given over an extended period.

Despite mixed results, the use of buserelin as a treatment for PMS symptoms remains promising. The study by Hammarbäck and Bäckström, with its larger sample size ($N = 23$) and double-blind, crossover design, is the best study model of the three, and its moderate buserelin dose seemed better tolerated while remaining effective in relieving symptoms.

The final method of ovulation suppression reviewed here is accomplished by surgical rather than pharmacologic means. Studies of oophorectomy and hysterectomy followed by a regimen of estrogen replacement indicated that this form of treatment eliminated mood and physical symptoms associated with PMS. Summaries of two such studies are found in Table 5–1. In studies by Casper and Hearn (1990) and Casson and colleagues (1990), women were selected on the basis of their unresponsiveness to previous medical therapy. In both studies, symptoms were recorded by using Reid's

Prospective Record of the Impact and Severity of Menstrual Symptomatology (PRISM) calendar (Reid 1985) for 2 months before and up to 1 year after surgery.

Overall, suppression of ovulation can effectively treat severe physical and affective symptoms of PMS. Although both pharmacologic and surgical treatments produce desired results, pharmacologic treatments are more desirable, because they allow for ovulation suppression through less radical means with essentially the same effect as surgery and with the reversibility not afforded by a surgical procedure.

Progesterone and Dydrogesterone

Several studies have tested the efficacy of progesterone, as well as that of its optical isomer, dydrogesterone, for the treatment of PMS symptoms. The details of these studies can be found in Table 5–2. A total of eight progesterone studies are reviewed here, all of which were designed in a double-blind, crossover manner. In all but two studies, treatment was administered by vaginal suppository. The doses in these six studies ranged from 200 to 800 mg daily, whereas doses in the two oral-treatment studies were either unreported (Dennerstein et al. 1985) or less than 10 mg daily (Jordheim 1972).

Of the eight studies reviewed, the most recent, by Freeman and colleagues (1990), also had the strongest study design. Subject selection was based on 2 months of prospective rating of symptoms followed by 2 months of placebo treatment, during which subjects continued to rate symptoms on a daily symptom report developed by the authors. Subjects were then randomly assigned to groups receiving either placebo or active treatment with progesterone, 400 or 800 mg daily. Each group continued treatment for 2 months, for a total of 6 months of double-blind, crossover treatment. Daily symptom reports, as well as subjects' global improvement ratings, showed no efficacy of progesterone at either dose. This result is in agreement with those of all other studies except that of Dennerstein and colleagues (1985), who found progesterone superior to placebo, but only in the first month. The study by

Table 5–2. Progesterone and dydrogesterone

Reference	Treatment	Measures	Methods	Results
Andersch and Hahn 1985	Progesterone	Modified CPRS scale	15 women; after 1-mo baseline, 100 mg vaginal progesterone or placebo twice daily, from 10 days before menses or at first symptoms, until menses onset, for 1 mo	No differences
Dennerstein et al. 1985	Progesterone	MDQ; BDI; STAI; MACL; daily symptom reports	23 women; oral active treatment or placebo (no doses given) for 2 mo	Progesterone clinically and statistically superior to placebo
Freeman et al. 1990	Progesterone	Daily symptom reports; patient global improvement ratings	121 women; 4-mo washout period, then randomized to groups receiving 400- and 800-mg progesterone suppositories daily for 2 mo; treatment on days 16–28 of each mo	No significant differences
Jordheim 1972	Progesterone (2.5 mg) + diuretic (2 mg)	Subjects' daily record	21 women; active treatment or placebo 3 times daily, from 10 days before menses, for 4 mo	No differences
Maddocks et al. 1986	Progesterone	BDI; Irritability Scale; STAI; MDQ, Form-T; PMTS Self-Rating Scale	20 women, 1-mo symptom rating; 400 mg vaginal progesterone or placebo daily from day 12 of cycle for 3 mo	No differences
Richter et al. 1984	Progesterone	Subjects' rankings of best cycles; authors' daily symptom rating scale	22 women assigned to treatment sequence consisting of 800 mg vaginal progesterone or placebo daily from day 15 to menses onset; 4 treatment cycles	No differences

Study	Treatment	Measure	Design	Results
Sampson 1979	Progesterone	MDQ; retrospective self-assessment	1-mo MDQ ratings; part 1: subjects ($n = 35$) received 400 mg progesterone or placebo daily for 1 mo; part 2: subjects ($n = 26$) received 800 mg progesterone or placebo daily for 1 mo	No preferences for either treatment
van der Meer et al. 1983	Progesterone	4-point symptom scale	13 women; 400 mg rectal progesterone or placebo daily, mid-cycle to menses onset, for 2 mo; gynecologist visit monthly	No differences
Dennerstein et al. 1986	Dydrogesterone	MDQ; STAI; MACL; daily symptom rating	24 women; 1-mo daily ratings, then 200 mg dydrogesterone or placebo daily on days 12–26 of each mo for 2 mo; women interviewed in menstrual period of each cycle	No differences, but treatment effect was noted
Kerr et al. 1980	Dydrogesterone	Gynecologist's assessment; plasma progesterone levels; symptom diaries	67 women; 20 mg active treatment or placebo daily on days 12–26 each mo in a single-blind trial for 6 mo	Subjects' diaries showed active treatment superior to placebo for 3 of 13 symptoms studied
Sampson et al. 1988	Dydrogesterone	MDQ	69 women; after 1-mo symptom rating, 20 mg dydrogesterone or placebo given daily, balanced, for 2 mo	No overall efficacy of dydrogesterone

Note. BDI = Beck Depression Inventory (Beck et al. 1979). CPRS = Comprehensive Psychopathological Rating Scale (Asberg et al. 1978). Irritability Scale: Buss and Durkee 1957. MACL = Mood Adjective Checklist (Mackay et al. 1978). MDQ = Menstrual Distress Questionnaire (Moos 1968). PMTS = Premenstrual Tension Syndrome (Haskett and Abplanalp 1983). STAI = State Trait Anxiety Inventory (Spielberger et al. 1970).

Dennerstein and colleagues (1985) had a much smaller sample size ($N = 23$) than did that by Freeman and colleagues (1990 [$N = 121$]), and it failed to report the progesterone dose tested. On the basis of this information and the negative results of the other six studies, progesterone cannot be recommended as a treatment for the symptoms of PMS.

Dydrogesterone, the optical isomer of progesterone, has also been studied as a possible treatment for PMS, and Table 5–2 reports the results of three such studies. Both Dennerstein and colleagues (1986) and Sampson and colleagues (1988) performed double-blind, crossover studies in which dydrogesterone (20 mg daily) was given during the luteal phase only. In addition, these two studies based diagnosis and treatment outcome on the Menstrual Distress Questionnaire (Moos 1968), which was completed by subjects on a daily basis. Neither study found dydrogesterone to be beneficial in the treatment of PMS. In a single-blind, placebo-controlled study, Kerr and colleagues (1980) also administered dydrogesterone at a dose of 20 mg daily on a cyclical basis (days 12–26 each month). This study, however, lacked prospective rating of symptoms to confirm the diagnosis of PMS, although subjects did keep daily symptom diaries during the treatment phase of the study. Gynecologists' assessments showed no clear efficacy of active treatment, and individuals' diaries showed dydrogesterone to be superior to placebo for very few symptoms. On the basis of the group means for the hormonal studies discussed here, the use of progesterone and dydrogesterone for the treatment of PMS does not appear to be beneficial.

Nutritional Supplements

A third group of studies (Table 5–3) concentrated on the efficacies of various nutritional supplements for the alleviation of the symptoms of PMS. In general, the bulk of these studies (7 of 14) were concerned with vitamin B6 (pyridoxine), but other nutrients, such as vitamin E, calcium, and evening primrose oil, as well as a nutrient combination called Optivite, have been studied.

The studies of vitamin B6 include a double-blind, crossover

Table 5–3. Nutritional supplements

Reference	Treatment	Measures	Methods	Results
London et al. 1987	α-Tocopherol	Questionnaire based on symptom classification of Steiner et al. (1980a) and Abraham (1984)	400 IU ($n = 22$) or placebo ($n = 19$) given for 3 mo; symptoms in follicular and luteal phases rated in all cycles	Active treatment superior to placebo in 3 of 4 Abraham categories and Steiner symptoms, but not at $P < .05$.
Thys-Jacobs et al. 1989	Calcium	Daily symptom scores; retrospective global assessment	33 women; 1,000 mg calcium carbonate or placebo daily for 3 mo, then a 4th mo of symptom scoring	Calcium superior to placebo
Callender et al. 1988	Evening primrose oil + vitamin supplement	Daily symptom diary; BDI; Salkind Inventory; Subjective report	10 women; 3,000 mg Efamol + Efavit (750 mg ascorbic acid, 30 mg zinc sulfate, and 150 mg each niacin and vitamin B6) or placebo, from day 7 to day 1 of menses, for 2 mo, with washout between	Subjective improvement in 70% of active treatment and 30% of placebo cycles; no differences in Beck or Salkind scores
Khoo et al. 1990	Evening primrose oil	4-point rating scale of symptoms	38 women met authors' criteria for PMS based on 1-mo symptom rating; Efamol or placebo given for 3 mo	No significant differences between treatments
Stephenson et al. 1988	Evening primrose oil + vitamin E	MDQ	70 women; 2-mo symptom rating; 8 capsules daily, active treatment or placebo, for 3 mo; monthly visit to nurse; MDQs completed 3 days/week	No differences between treatments

(continued)

Table 5–3. Nutritional supplements (*continued*)

Reference	Treatment	Measures	Methods	Results
Chakmakjian et al. 1985	Optivite	MSD; self-rating of symptoms	Subjects (*n* = 31) took 6 tablets of Optivite or placebo daily for 3 cycles; MSD completed in wks 2 and 4 of all cycles	16 subjects preferred Optivite, 7 preferred placebo, 8 had no preference; MSD scores lower for PMT-A and PMT-C on Optivite
Stewart 1987	Optivite	Self-rating of symptoms	3 mo of Optivite or placebo; 4 tablets/day in 1st 2 wks, then 8 tablets/day (*n* = 119); or 2 tablets/day in 1st 2 wks, then 4 tablets/day (*n* = 104)	Optivite superior to placebo only in high-dose trial
Abraham and Hargrove 1980	Pyridoxine	MSD; daily weight records	25 women; 500 mg pyridoxine or placebo daily for 3 mo; daily weight and MSD ratings	Pyridoxine superior in 22 subjects, as shown by MSD score
Barr 1984	Pyridoxine	Daily symptom records	48 women; 200 mg pyridoxine or placebo daily, from cycle day 10 to day 3 of menses, for 2 mo	Pyridoxine superior to placebo
Hagen et al. 1985	Pyridoxine	Global VAS; self-rating of symptoms; plasma magnesium	Subjects (*n* = 34) received 100 mg pyridoxine or placebo daily for 2 mo; VAS completed at end of each 2-mo period	Treatments equivalent; order effect observed

Study	Treatment	Measures	Sample/Dosing	Results
Harrison et al. 1984	Pyridoxine	Physician's CGI; PAF; daily self-rating scale	Placebo nonresponders ($n = 20$) given 50–150 mg pyridoxine + 1.5–6.0 g L-tryptophan daily for 3 mo	No differences between treatments
Kendall and Schnurr 1987	Pyridoxine	Daily symptom records; PAF; MDQ, Form-T	55 women; 150 mg pyridoxine or placebo daily for 2 mo; daily MDQ and symptom records	Pyridoxine superior to placebo for autonomic and behavioral symptoms only
Malmgren et al. 1987	Pyridoxine	Platelet serotonin uptake	300 mg pyridoxine or placebo daily, from cycle day 15 to day 1 of menses, for 2 mo	No differences between treatments
Williams et al. 1985	Pyridoxine	Investigator's final assessment; daily record of tablets taken and symptom severity	50–200 mg pyridoxine ($n = 204$) or placebo ($n = 230$) for 3 cycles	No difference in individual symptoms, but overall results showed pyridoxine superior to placebo

Note. BDI = Beck Depression Inventory (Beck et al. 1979). CGI = Clinical Global Impressions Scale. MDQ = Menstrual Distress Questionnaire (Moos 1968). MSQ = Menstrual Symptom Questionnaire (Abraham 1980). PAF = Premenstrual Assessment Form (Endicott et al. 1986). PMT-A and PMT-C = Premenstrual Tension Syndrome—Subtype A and Premenstrual Tension Syndrome—Subtype C (Abraham 1980). VAS = visual analog scale.

study in which vitamin B_6 was given in a daily dose of 500 mg (Abraham and Hargrove 1980). They used their menstrual symptom questionnaire as an outcome measure. In this study, active treatment was superior to placebo for 22 of 25 women. Based on the subjects' daily records of symptoms, Barr (1984) found a cyclical (i.e., administered from cycle day 10 to day 3 of menses), 200-mg daily dose of vitamin B_6 to be superior to placebo. This study, however, did not require prospective confirmation of premenstrual symptoms before subject selection. The third study supporting the use of vitamin B_6 was performed by Williams and colleagues (1985) in a placebo-controlled, double-blind manner. The results of this study were based on subjects' diary cards, which provided a record of the number of tablets taken and the severity of symptoms experienced. Subjects' compliance, however, in completing and returning these cards was rather low—only half of all cards were turned in, and many were incomplete. Another complicating factor in this study was evidence of a dose effect; improvement was more likely when the number of tablets taken increased, regardless of the treatment given.

London and colleagues (1987) studied vitamin E (α-tocopherol). In this randomized, double-blind study, 22 subjects received active treatment (400 IU daily) and 19 subjects received placebo for 3 months. Treatment outcome for the study was based on a questionnaire that included symptoms classified by Steiner and colleagues (1980a), as well as those in the four symptom categories of Abraham (1980). Results of the vitamin E study showed it to be superior to placebo clinically, though not statistically, for the relief of PMS. No side effects were reported for vitamin E, but one woman taking placebo did report headache, chest pain, anxiety, and paranoid ideation.

A double-blind, crossover study by Thys-Jacobs and colleagues (1989) demonstrated the efficacy of calcium (1,000 mg daily) for the treatment of PMS. Documentation of symptoms before, during, and 1 month after treatment was facilitated by daily symptom questionnaires. Subjects ($N = 33$) also rated treatment preference retrospectively. Calcium was superior to placebo. Side effects such as nausea, constipation, flatulence, and gastrointestinal discomfort were noted with the active treatment.

Another nutritional supplement studied was evening primrose oil (Efamol), which contains γ-linolenic acid, a derivative of *cis*-linoleic acid and a critical precursor of prostaglandin E_1. Levels of *cis*-linoleic acid have been reported to be higher in women with PMS than in control subjects but with reduced metabolites, suggesting a low conversion rate of *cis*-linoleic acid to γ-linolenic acid (Brush 1984). Administration of γ-linolenic acid by means of evening primrose oil was thought to be capable of overcoming any block in prostaglandin E_1 production. Although Callender and colleagues (1988) reported subjective improvement during 70% of cycles in which active treatment was given and only 30% of those in which placebo was given, they found no differences in other outcome measures. This lack of treatment efficacy was more clearly demonstrated in studies by Khoo and colleagues (1990) and Stephenson and colleagues (1988). The weight of evidence from these three double-blind, crossover studies suggests that evening primrose oil is not an effective treatment for PMS symptoms.

Two efficacy studies of Optivite, a multivitamin, multimineral supplement, have provided mixed results for PMS treatment. Chakmakjian and colleagues (1985) performed a double-blind, crossover study of Optivite (six tablets daily) and placebo therapy. No clear efficacy of the active treatment was indicated in this study (Table 5–3). Stewart (1987), in a random, double-blind study, suggested that Optivite is efficacious at a relatively high dose (eight tablets daily) but not at a lower dose (four tablets daily). The results of both of these studies suggest that perhaps a third study, using at least eight tablets daily, would help to answer the question of the efficacy of Optivite for the treatment of PMS. Double-blind replication studies are needed to determine unequivocally whether any of these nutrient supplements are more effective than placebo for treating LLPDD.

Diuretics

The use of diuretics in the treatment of PMS has been extensively studied, primarily in the past. Table 5–4 lists the various

Table 5–4. Diuretics

Reference	Treatment	Measures	Methods	Results
Hoffman 1979	Ammonium chloride + caffeine	Weight records, days 14–17, 18–23, and 24	22 women, 1,950 mg ammonium chloride + 600 mg of caffeine or placebo daily on cycle days 18–24	Diuretic superior to placebo
Andersch and Hahn 1982	Bromocriptine	Plasma progesterone, prolactin; self-rating; physical symptoms	35 women; 2.5 mg bromocriptine daily for 3 mo or placebo daily for 1 mo, from symptom onset; blood samples in luteal phase of each cycle	Bromocriptine superior for reducing finger and leg swelling; no other differences
Andersen et al. 1977	Bromocriptine	Self-rating of symptoms; plasma progesterone, prolactin, and estradiol	21 women; 5.0 mg bromocriptine or placebo daily, from day of expected ovulation to menses onset; symptoms rated on cycle days 7–26	No difference between treatments
Benedek-Jaszmann and Sturtevant 1976	Bromocriptine	Plasma prolactin, FSH, LH, estradiol, and progesterone; urinary potassium, sodium, creatinine	10 women; 5.0 mg bromocriptine or placebo daily for 1 cycle, from day 10 until menstruation	Bromocriptine superior for physical and mood symptoms; no effect on creatinine; increased sodium and potassium excretion
Ghose and Coppen 1977	Bromocriptine	MSQ	13 women; 1.5 mg bromocriptine or placebo daily, from 10 days before menses onset	No difference between treatments

Graham et al. 1978	Bromocriptine	Daily record of body weight, breast size, and basal body temperature; daily symptom rating	8 women; 2.5 mg bromocriptine daily, days 14–16, and 5.0 mg/day until menstruation, or placebo daily, for 2 mo	Bromocriptine improved bloating and psychiatric symptoms; no changes in other physical symptoms
Kullander and Svanberg 1979	Bromocriptine	Self-rating of symptoms; plasma estradiol, FSH, LH, progesterone, and prolactin	10 women; 5 mg bromocriptine or placebo daily, from day 14 until menstruation, for 2 mo	No treatment differences for symptom relief; bromocriptine reduced prolactin levels and increased FSH and LH
Steiner et al. 1983	Bromocriptine	VAS; MDQ; MAACL; STAI; Hamilton Rating Scale for Depression; Carroll Depression Scale	2.5 ($n = 8$), 5.0 ($n = 8$), or 7.5 ($n = 8$) mg bromocriptine or placebo ($n = 6$) daily for 3 consecutive mo; physician visits on days 9 and 26 each mo	No difference between treatments
Ylostalo et al. 1982	Bromocriptine	Daily weight records; subject symptom ratings	2.5–5 mg bromocriptine or placebo ($n = 18$), or 5–10 mg norethisterone daily from day 12 to menses onset; placebo in cycles 1 and 4, active treatment in cycles 2 and 3	Bromocriptine superior to placebo and norethisterone, but norethisterone better tolerated

(continued)

Table 5–4. Diuretics *(continued)*

Reference	Treatment	Measures	Methods	Results
Mattsson and von Schoultz 1974	Lithium or chlorthalidone	Physician's symptom ratings; subject symptom ratings	18 women; 25 mg chlorthalidone daily in wk 1, then 50 mg daily, or placebo; 24 mEq/day in 2 premenstrual wks	No difference between treatments
Werch and Kane 1976	Metolazone	Body weight; self-rating of symptoms	1.0 ($n = 13$), 2.5 ($n = 15$), and 5.0 ($n = 5$) mg metolazone daily; excessive diuresis at 5-mg dose, so switched to a lower dose	Less weight gain in diuretic cycles; less water retention and negative affect as well
O'Brien et al. 1979	Spironolactone	PMI (luteal VAS–follicular VAS score)	18 women; 100 mg spironolactone or placebo daily on days 18–26 for at least 1 mo	Spironolactone superior to placebo on PMI
Vellacott et al. 1987	Spironolactone	Daily weight records; daily symptom records; plasma hormone levels; urinary aldosterone	100 mg spironolactone ($n = 31$) or placebo ($n = 32$) daily, from day 12 to menses onset, for 2 mo; blood sample on day 21 of each cycle	Spironolactone superior to placebo on many symptoms, but none reached significance; no other differences between treatments

Note. FSH = follicle-stimulating hormone. HRSD = Hamilton Rating Scale for Depression (Hamilton 1960). LH = luteinizing hormone. MAACL = Multiple Affect Adjective Check List (Zuckerman and Lubin 1965). MDQ = Menstrual Distress Questionnaire (Moos 1968). MSQ = Menstrual Symptom Questionnaire (Abraham 1980). PMI = Premenstrual Mood Index. STAI = State Trait Anxiety Inventory (Spielberger et al. 1970). VAS = visual analog scale. Carroll Depression Scale (Carroll et al. 1981).

diuretics included in this review. Although bromocriptine has been the focus of most of this research, its efficacy remains unclear. Bromocriptine is a dopamine agonist that has been proposed to exert its effects by inhibiting the release of prolactin and stimulating the excretion of electrolytes, causing diuresis (Kullander and Svanberg 1979).

All but two of the eight studies of bromocriptine described here were performed in a double-blind, crossover manner; the other two (Steiner et al. 1983; Ylostalo et al. 1982) were designed as placebo-controlled trials. In every study but that by Steiner and colleagues (1983), the medication dosage ranged from 2.5 to 5.0 mg daily, and administration was limited to the luteal phase of each cycle. Results of studies by Andersen and colleagues (1977), Ghose and Coppen (1977), Kullander and Svanberg (1979), and Steiner and colleagues (1983) revealed no differences between bromocriptine and placebo. Other studies, by Andersch and Hahn (1982), Benedek-Jaszmann and Sturtevant (1976), Graham and colleagues (1978), and Ylostalo and colleagues (1982), produced mixed results, with only a few symptoms alleviated by the active treatment. On the basis of this information, it seems that at best, bromocriptine is only partially effective at reducing the symptoms of PMS, most often exerting relief only for breast symptoms. This particular diuretic, then, holds little promise as a treatment for other symptoms of PMS.

Hoffman (1979) reported on the efficacy of ammonium chloride (1,950 mg daily) plus caffeine (600 mg daily) in a double-blind, crossover study. This study concentrated on weight gain as the primary symptom of interest. Diuretic was superior to placebo for reduction of premenstrual weight gain, but no mention was made regarding the relief of any mood or other physical symptoms. For the time being, then, this treatment may be considered effective for only a small part of the overall PMS symptomatology.

Mattsson and von Schoultz (1974) carried out a double-blind, crossover study in which chlorthalidone (25–50 mg daily), lithium carbonate (24 mg daily), and placebo were compared. Prospective daily rating was not a part of this study; rather, women and their physicians made independent ratings of symptoms once during the luteal phase of each cycle. According to these ratings, all treatments improved all symptoms. In fact, more women preferred placebo than lithium or chlorthalidone. Another finding of interest was that the diuretic effect of lithium observed in this study was not seen when women took chlorthalidone, a well-known diuretic.

Metolazone in various doses was studied by Werch and Kane (1976). In this double-blind, crossover study, body weight was the primary outcome measure, but subjects ($N = 46$) also rated several other symptoms, both physical and affective. Once again, prospective ratings were not made on a daily basis; rather, symptoms were rated during bimonthly physician visits. At the end of treatment, subjects receiving metolazone at all doses showed significant improvement of symptoms when compared with placebo. In addition, the lower doses of metolazone seemed equally as effective as the higher doses, but without side effects such as excessive diuresis and weakness.

The final diuretic discussed here is spironolactone, and the results of two studies of this drug are shown in Table 5–4. In both studies, conducted in a double-blind manner, spironolactone (100 mg daily) or placebo was administered during the luteal phase of each cycle. O'Brien and colleagues (1979) found spironolactone to be superior to placebo on the basis of a premenstrual mood index, which was calculated from daily visual analog scales of symptom severity. Vellacott and colleagues (1987) found that, although spironolactone was generally more effective than placebo for the relief of PMS symptoms, this relief failed to reach statistical significance for any symptom but bloating. It thus appears that diuretics, in general, should be considered as possible treatments for PMS, especially for premenstrual bloating or weight gain.

Psychopharmacologic Agents

Several studies have examined the efficacy of psychopharmacologic treatment of PMS. Table 5–5 shows the various anxiolytic agents and antidepressants included in this review.

The anxiolytic alprazolam was the focus of three recent studies, in all of which treatment was administered only during the luteal

Table 5–5. Psychopharmacologic agents

Reference	Treatment	Measures	Methods	Results
Harrison et al. 1987	Alprazolam	CGI; GAS	34 women; 0.25–4 mg alprazolam or placebo daily, from symptom onset to menses onset, for 3 mo, with tapering of drug	Alprazolam superior to placebo
Harrison et al. 1990	Alprazolam	CGI; GAS; DRF; PAF	30 women; 0.5–4 mg alprazolam or placebo daily from symptom onset to menses onset, for 3 mo, with tapering of drug; PAF completed at end of each cycle	Alprazolam superior to placebo
Smith et al. 1987	Alprazolam	Daily symptom diary	14 women; 0.75 mg alprazolam or placebo daily, from cycle day 20 through day 2 of menses, for 2 mo, with tapering of drug	Alprazolam superior to placebo
Rickels et al. 1989	Buspirone	Daily symptom diary	Placebo nonresponders assigned to 20 mg buspirone ($n = 17$) or placebo ($n = 17$) daily during the last 12 days of cycle for 3 mo	Buspirone superior to placebo
Eriksson et al. 1990	Clomipramine	VAS; subject ratings	Placebo nonresponders ($n = 5$) given 25–50 mg clomipramine daily for 5 cycles; symptoms rated daily	Clomipramine superior to placebo
Sundblad et al. 1992	Clomipramine	VAS	Subjects assigned to 3 treatment cycles of either 25–75 mg clomipramine ($n = 20$) or placebo ($n = 20$) daily	Clomipramine superior to placebo in reducing irritability and dysphoria

(continued)

Table 5–5. Psychopharmacologic agents (*continued*)

Reference	Treatment	Measures	Methods	Results
Rickels et al. 1990	Fluoxetine	Daily Symptom Rating Scale; HRSD	10 women; 1-mo rating, then 1 mo on placebo, and 20 mg fluoxetine daily for at least 2 mo; 10 women in placebo control group	Fluoxetine superior to placebo
Stone et al. 1991	Fluoxetine	DRF; GAS	20 mg fluoxetine ($n = 9$) or placebo ($n = 6$) daily for 2 mo; clinic visit in each luteal phase for GAS	Fluoxetine superior to placebo
Singer et al. 1974	Lithium	Global Clinical Scale; Target Symptoms Scale; self-rating scale	14 women; 750–1,000 mg lithium carbonate or placebo daily, with target blood level of drug of 0.8–1.3 mEq/L	No differences between treatments
Steiner et al. 1980b	Lithium	VAS; MDQ; MACL; STAI; CDS	15 women; 600–900 mg lithium carbonate daily, after a no-treatment baseline cycle	Efficacy of lithium not shown
Harrison et al. 1989	Nortriptyline	DRF; PAF; CGI	11 women; 50–125 mg nortriptyline daily, given to placebo nonresponders	Nortriptyline superior to placebo in 8 of 11 subjects

Note. CDS = Carroll Depression Scale (Carroll et al. 1981). CGI = Clinical Global Impressions Scale. DRF = Daily Rating Form (Endicott et al. 1986). GAS = Global Assessment Scale (Endicott et al 1976). HRSD = Hamilton Rating Scale for Depression (Hamilton 1960). MACL = Mood Adjective Checklist (Mackay et al. 1978). MDQ = Menstrual Distress Questionnaire (Moos 1968). PAF = Premenstrual Assessment Form (Endicott et al. 1986). STAI = State Trait Anxiety Inventory (Spielberger et al. 1970). VAS = visual analog scale.

phase of each cycle. Harrison and colleagues (1987, 1990) performed two double-blind, crossover studies of alprazolam at doses ranging from 0.25 to 4 mg daily. Smith and colleagues (1987) used an alprazolam dose of 0.75 mg daily, also in a double-blind, crossover study. In all three studies, subject selection was based on at least 1 month of prospective ratings of symptoms to confirm the diagnosis of PMS, and symptom rating was continued throughout the treatment phase in all studies. The results of these studies confirm the superiority of alprazolam over placebo for relief of PMS symptoms. Treatment in all cases was tapered off at the end of each month in order to avoid withdrawal symptoms.

Buspirone is another anxiolytic found to be efficacious as a treatment for PMS. Treatment in a study by Rickels and colleagues (1989) was, as in the alprazolam studies, given only during the luteal phase of each menstrual cycle. The medication dose in this placebo-controlled, double-blind study was 20 mg daily. Although buspirone seems promising for the treatment of PMS, more studies on its efficacy are necessary to support the findings discussed here.

Clomipramine is among the antidepressants that have been studied as a treatment for PMS. Details of a study by Eriksson and colleagues (1990) are shown in Table 5–5. In this study, subjects who responded to placebo were screened out, and those who did not were treated with clomipramine (25–50 mg daily). Visual analog scales of symptoms showed clomipramine to be superior to placebo for the above dose range, that is, lower than the dose generally used in the treatment of depression. Still, this study had only five subjects, making replication with a larger sample desirable. Side effects such as sedation, constipation, and dry mouth were reported, even at this relatively low dose of clomipramine. In a study by Sundblad and colleagues (1992), subjects were assigned to three treatment cycles of clomipramine (25–75 mg daily) or placebo. As in the study by Eriksson and colleagues (1990), symptom ratings were made on a visual analog scale. Active treatment was found to be superior to placebo in this particular study as well, but only a few symptoms were monitored.

The results of two studies of fluoxetine, another antidepressant, are shown in Table 5–5. Both Rickels and colleagues (1990) and Stone and colleagues (1991) found fluoxetine (20 mg daily) to be superior to placebo for relief of PMS. In both studies, prospective ratings for at least 1 month were used as a means of selecting subjects who met DSM-III-R criteria for LLPDD. Although fluoxetine was found to be a beneficial treatment for PMS, some side effects (nausea, insomnia, headache, dizziness, nervousness, increased appetite, and decreased libido) were noted.

The antidepressant nortriptyline was the subject of a study by Harrison and colleagues (1989). Only subjects who showed no previous response to placebo ($N = 11$) were selected for this open study, and their symptoms met DSM-III-R criteria for LLPDD for 2 months before treatment. Nortriptyline in doses of 50–125 mg daily was effective in 8 of the 11 women participating in the study. As is the case with other promising treatments, replication with a larger sample, possibly in a double-blind, crossover manner, is desirable.

Of all the psychopharmacologic agents discussed here, only lithium has been shown to be ineffective as a treatment for PMS. Studies by Singer and colleagues (1974) and Steiner and colleagues (1980b) showed no benefit of lithium at doses ranging from 600 to 1,000 mg daily. On the basis of these findings and the high frequency of side effects (nausea, tremor, dizziness), lithium is not recommended for the treatment of PMS.

In summary, most of the anxiolytic and antidepressant agents discussed here have been shown to be beneficial in the treatment of PMS. Only lithium has been shown to be ineffective for this purpose. There remains, however, a need to replicate studies of treatments such as buspirone and nortriptyline.

Melatonin Inhibitors

Table 5–6 lists studies of treatments intended to suppress secretion of melatonin. Included in this group are bright light, atenolol, and propranolol.

Bright light tends to suppress melatonin secretion in early evening, with a rebound later in the night, whereas atenolol and propranolol are β-adrenergic agonists that suppress melatonin

Table 5–6. Melatonin inhibition

Reference	Treatment	Measures	Methods	Results
Parry et al. 1991	Atenolol	HRSD; VAS	11 women; 100 mg atenolol or placebo daily, 7 days before menses, for 1 mo	Atenolol not superior to placebo
Rausch et al. 1988	Atenolol	MDQ; BDI; Steiner rating scale; HRSD; POMS	16 women; 2-mo symptom rating before treatment, with DSM-III-R criteria met; 50 mg atenolol or placebo daily, from 10 days before menses, for 1 mo	Trend toward lower symptom scores on atenolol, but not significant on most measures
Parry et al. 1987	Light, propranolol, or atenolol	HRSD; blood melatonin	1 woman; LLPDD in fall and winter; 4 trials: 1) 2,500 lux daily, from symptom onset; 2) light plus placebo or melatonin (1.6 mg), or placebo alone; 3) propranolol (40 mg) or placebo, then 1 mo at half dose; 4) atenolol or placebo, 1 mo each	All 3 forms of treatment superior to placebo
Parry et al. 1989	Light	HRSD; BDI; VAS	6 women; 2,500 lux, 2 h daily in morning and evening, from 7 days before to menses onset, for 1 mo	Only evening light significantly improved symptoms

Note. BDI = Beck Depression Inventory (Beck et al. 1979). HRSD = Hamilton Rating Scale for Depression (Hamilton 1960). MDQ = Menstrual Distress Questionnaire (Moos 1968). POMS = Profile of Mood States (McNair et al. 1971). VAS = visual analog scale. Steiner rating scale: Steiner et al. 1980a.

secretion throughout the night. Parry and colleagues (1987) first took on this research with a study of a 24-year-old woman with a history of LLPDD only in fall and winter. She underwent four different treatment trials (Table 5–6), the first of which tested the efficacy of phototherapy presented daily from 6:00 P.M. to 11:00 P.M. during luteal phases. In a second trial, the subject was treated first with light plus placebo and then with light plus melatonin to determine whether melatonin would reverse the therapeutic effect of light. As predicted, oral administration of melatonin was found to reverse the therapeutic effect of light. The third trial was a double-blind, crossover study in which the subject received propranolol (40 mg) or placebo nightly during the luteal phase, with a subsequent cycle of treatment at half the original dose. In the fourth trial, atenolol (50 mg daily) was given for 1 month, followed by 1 month of placebo. The outcome of all four trials was based on weekly scores on the Hamilton Rating Scale for Depression (Hamilton 1960). For this particular woman, all three active treatments (bright light, atenolol, and propranolol) were found to be beneficial in the relief of depressive symptoms during the luteal phase.

Parry and colleagues (1989) later reported the results of a randomized, crossover trial of morning versus evening light (2,500 lux). Six women met DSM-III-R criteria for LLPDD and entered the study. Light therapy was presented in 2-hour sessions during the luteal phase, with Hamilton (1960) and Beck (1979) measures taken at the end of each luteal phase. The results of this study showed that, although there were no significant differences between morning and evening light therapy, the evening treatment was more promising, significantly improving Hamilton scores and nearly improving Beck scores.

A double-blind, crossover study of atenolol (50 mg daily) was carried out by Rausch and colleagues (1988). The 16 women in the study were accepted only after meeting DSM-III-R criteria for LLPDD. Outcome measures employed included the Menstrual Distress Questionnaire (Moos 1968), the Profile of Mood States (McNair et al. 1971), the Beck Depression Inventory (Beck et al. 1979), and the Hamilton Rating Scale for Depression. Statistically significant changes were noted in only a few symptom items (vigor, friendliness, irritability). In view of the numerous outcome measures used and the large number of comparisons made, such results could be due to chance factors alone. The authors concluded that a larger dose may be necessary to produce a measurable therapeutic effect, but the results of a later study (Parry et al. 1991) of atenolol cast doubt on this assumption. In this double-blind, crossover study, 11 women with LLPDD were given 100 mg of atenolol or placebo daily during the symptomatic luteal phase. There was no significant improvement noted after treatment, as measured by the Hamilton Rating Scale for Depression.

One possible explanation for the conflicting findings in this area is that melatonin may be implicated only in seasonal forms of LLPDD (Parry et al. 1991). This would limit the usefulness of melatonin-inhibiting therapies to such cases. Bright-light treatment, however, may produce results via mechanisms other than melatonin inhibition. Placebo-controlled studies of bright-light treatment are needed for clarification, but pharmacologic methods of suppressing melatonin secretion do not yet appear to be promising treatments for LLPDD.

Parry and colleagues (1991) studied 11 women with prospectively diagnosed premenstrual depression. In a double-blind, crossover trial, the women were given atenolol (100 mg daily) or placebo for 1 week before the anticipated onset of the next menses. The authors found no statistically significant effects of atenolol compared with placebo on daily mood ratings or on sleep variables.

The treatment of PMS by melatonin inhibition has shown mixed results, as shown in the studies discussed here. One problem presented by the light studies is the lack of placebo-control conditions. The best solution in this case would be replicating these studies while maintaining stringent subject selection. As for pharmacologic treatments, replication with larger sample sizes in double-blind, crossover studies is desirable.

Miscellaneous Somatic Treatments

Several studies of PMS treatments were not appropriate for inclusion within the various categories discussed thus far. Many of these treatments have been supported by noteworthy research. Details of these studies can be found in Table 5–7.

Clonidine, which decreases the amount of norepinephrine released at presynaptic sites, was studied by Giannini and colleagues (1988). In this 4-month, double-blind, crossover study, the efficacy of clonidine (17 mg/kg daily) was demonstrated, based on luteal phase scores on the Brief Psychiatric Rating Scale (Overall and Gorham 1962). Although results were encouraging, the outcome measure tracked only psychiatric symptoms, and no mention was made of any physical symptom measure. Another complicating factor was selection of women with PMS symptoms, but no mention of any particular selection criteria. Further study, using more extensive outcome measures and appropriate selection criteria, is recommended if clonidine is to be considered a valid treatment for PMS.

Toth and colleagues (1988) studied the effects of an antibiotic, doxycycline, on symptoms of PMS. An infectious etiology was proposed for some cases of PMS (subclinical endometrial or ovarian infection), and it was deemed possible that doxycycline could clear up such infections and relieve PMS symptoms. Women received doxycycline (200 mg daily [$n = 15$]) or placebo ($n = 15$) for 2 months in this double-blind study. Based on scores from visual analog scales, doxycycline was significantly more effective than placebo at relieving PMS symptoms, even up to 6 months after treatment had ceased. The problem with this study was methodological. It deserves replication in a carefully selected sample of women with prospectively confirmed LLPDD.

Results of three double-blind, crossover studies and one double-blind, placebo-controlled trial of mefenamic acid are shown in Table 5–7. This agent appears to act as a prostaglandin inhibitor in the relief of PMS. All four of the studies of mefenamic acid agreed that this treatment was superior to placebo for the relief of premenstrual pain. Treatment in all cases was given in the luteal phase of each cycle, generally at the onset of symptoms. The medication doses in the studies ranged from 750 mg daily (Gunston 1986) to 2,000 mg daily (Jakubowicz et al. 1984; Mira et al. 1986). In the two higher-dose studies, side effects such as nausea, skin rash, and di-

Table 5–7. Miscellaneous treatments

Reference	Treatment	Measures	Methods	Results
Giannini et al. 1988	Clonidine	Brief Psychiatric Rating Scale	24 women; 17 mg clonidine or placebo daily for 2 mo	Clonidine superior to placebo
Toth et al. 1988	Doxycycline	VAS; Menstrual Flow Questionnaire	1-mo baseline; 200 mg doxycycline ($n = 15$) or placebo ($n = 15$) daily for 2 mo; 6-mo follow-up visit	Doxycycline superior to placebo at 6-mo follow-up
Gunston 1986	Mefenamic acid	Daily symptom checklist; subjective assessment	42 women; 1-mo baseline, then 750 mg mefenamic acid or placebo daily, days 11–26, for 4 mo	Mefenamic acid superior to placebo according to subjective assessment
Jakubowicz 1984	Mefenamic acid	Daily symptom checklist	80 women in open trial, 19 in double-blind crossover study; 1,500–2,000 mg mefenamic acid or placebo daily	Mefenamic acid superior to placebo
Mira et al. 1986	Mefenamic acid	VAS (mood); questionnaire (physical)	15 women; 3-mo rating, then 1,000–2,000 mg mefenamic acid or placebo daily	Mefenamic acid superior for most symptoms
Wood and Jakubowicz 1980	Mefenamic acid	Daily symptom checklist; subjective performance	37 women; 1-mo baseline, then 1,500 mg mefenamic acid or placebo daily, from symptom onset, for 1 mo	Mefenamic acid superior to placebo according to subjective reports
Chuong et al. 1988	Naltrexone	MDQ; basal body temperature; daily diary	20 women; 2 no-treatment cycles, then 50 mg naltrexone or placebo daily for 3 mo, followed by 1 mo of no treatment and 3 mo of alternative treatment	Naltrexone superior to placebo
Nikolai et al. 1990	L-Thyroxine	MSD	15 no-treatment control subjects and 44 PMS subjects; 2-mo rating, then PMS subjects given 1.6 μg L-thyroxine per kg or placebo for 2 mo	No differences between treatments

Note. MDQ = Menstrual Distress Questionnaire (Moos 1968). MSD = Menstrual Symptom Diary (Abraham 1980). VAS = visual analog scale. Brief Psychiatric Rating Scale (Overall and Gorham 1962). Menstrual Flow Questionnaire (Macleod Laboratory, New York Hospital–Cornell Medical Center).

arrhea were reported. Mefenamic acid appears to be effective as a cyclically administered treatment for premenstrual pain, even at half the maximum dose (2,000 mg daily) used here, but side effects of treatment are considerable.

Chuong and colleagues (1988) reported the results of a double-blind crossover study of naltrexone, a narcotic agonist that does not appear to have any addiction or withdrawal risks. Daily diaries and Menstrual Distress Questionnaires (Moos 1968) demonstrated the superiority of cyclic administration of naltrexone (50 mg daily) over placebo for symptom relief. Some side effects reported at this dose were nausea, decreased appetite, and dizziness, which the authors suggested may be reduced by decreasing or dividing the medication dose. Study replication, perhaps at a lower medication dose, is recommended in the case of this treatment.

Nikolai and colleagues (1990) performed a double-blind, placebo-controlled study of L-thyroxine as a possible treatment for PMS, following a suggestion that some form of thyroid hypofunction may be at least partly responsible for the appearance of PMS symptoms. After 2 months of treating subjects with either L-thyroxine ($1.6 \mu g/kg$ [$n = 22$]) or placebo ($n = 22$), the authors found no benefit of L-thyroxine, as shown by the Menstrual Symptom Diary (Abraham 1980).

There has been considerable discussion in the literature of oral contraceptives as a means of ameliorating both premenstrual and menstrual complaints. As of this writing (1991), however, there have been no published studies that include appropriate subject selection criteria, random assignment, or placebo-control subjects. For this reason, the use of oral contraceptives has been omitted from this discussion.

Psychosocial Treatments

Because many symptoms common to PMS are emotional or have been amenable to psychosocial intervention, psychotherapy and strategies to change behavior are often suggested as a form of treatment. Recommended interventions range from intensive psychotherapy to self-management strategies such as dietary modification (Table 5–8). The efficacy of these approaches, however, has rarely been subjected to a stringent test. Because of the relative scarcity of published reports in scientific journals, we also searched the dissertation literature for relevant studies to include in this review. Consistent with the previous section, we attempted to focus primarily on those studies that used some method of confirming a diagnosis of PMS or LLPDD and employed a placebo or comparison condition.

Insight-Oriented Psychotherapy

Very little research exists on the use of traditional forms of psychotherapy as treatment for menstrually related mood symptoms. Only two early works, by Rees (1953) and Fortin and colleagues (1958), reported on the use of insight-oriented individual therapy for women with self-diagnosed premenstrual complaints. Neither of these studies found evidence that favored the use of this treatment. These authors operated from the belief that PMS is influenced by unconscious motives or results from neurotic tendencies, consistent with traditional, dynamically oriented models of psychotherapy. Because of numerous

---

Table 5–8. Suggested psychosocial treatments for premenstrual syndrome

- Insight-oriented psychotherapy
- Marital/family therapy
- Relation therapy
- Biofeedback
- Anxiety/anger management
- Relaxation-emotive therapy
- Cognitive-behavior therapy
  Thought stopping
  Cognitive restructuring
  Covert reinforcement
- Support groups
- Self-hypnosis
- Physical exercise
- Assertiveness training
- Dietary modification
  Reduction of caffeine, refined sugar, salt
  Increased intake of complex carbohydrates
  Frequent feedings
- Stress management
  Problem solving
  Time management
  Self-monitoring

---

flaws in the design of these studies (one of which was uncontrolled), they will not be elaborated upon here. Clearly, the use of insight-oriented procedures needs careful evaluation.

Group Therapy

Supportive group therapy for women with PMS is thought to be helpful in decreasing women's isolation and providing new ways of coping with symptoms. One published study has attempted to evaluate the effect of group support. Walton and Youngkin (1987) examined changes in self-esteem after participation in a support group. Eleven subjects were diagnosed by examination of prospective ratings, and the five who accepted the invitation to participate in the group were later compared with those who declined and served as the comparison subjects. Most participants (81%) used other forms of treatment (progesterone, dietary changes) during the study, and members of the support group met with a PMS counselor once a week for 8 weeks. At the end of this period, no significant differences in self-esteem were noted between the comparison and support group. Failure to control for cycle phase when administering pre- and postintervention measures, however, may have influenced the results. The authors did not report on possible changes in symptoms in group members. The small size of the sample may have contributed to the lack of significant findings, but any results would be difficult to interpret because of the confounding influence of multiple treatments in this sample. It is noteworthy that group members differed from nonmembers with respect to the number of previous treatments suggested to them by professionals; thus, these subjects may have represented the more severe cases.

In the dissertation literature, support groups have been used as a comparison condition to measure the effect of nonspecific variables, such as contact with a therapist. The effectiveness of group support is then contrasted with an "active" treatment, such as relaxation training or cognitive techniques. Of three such studies, two found support groups to be as effective as cognitive-behavior therapy in reducing some symptoms (Reed 1986; Weiss 1988).

A study in which group cognitive-behavior therapy, a support group, and an assessment-only control group were compared, however, found that all were associated with similar reductions in the number and severity of symptoms at approximately 1 month after treatment (Margolis 1985). These three studies are superior in design to the two published articles, because subjects were randomized to conditions, preexisting treatments were controlled for, and specific diagnostic criteria for PMS were used.

Women generally report satisfaction with the group experience and feel they benefit personally from meeting and talking with other women who have similar problems. Actual improvement in symptoms has been demonstrated in only two of the controlled studies. Whether participation in a support group can bring about a sustained positive outcome, however, has not been evaluated, because studies have not included long-term follow-up. Since the content and structure of so-called "support" groups vary greatly, the potency of this treatment may depend on whether other psychotherapeutic elements, such as problem-solving or specific suggestions regarding life-style changes, are included.

Cognitive-Behavior and Self-Management Techniques

Cognitive-behavior techniques have also been suggested as a treatment for PMS, because negative attributions and interpretation of events can lead to or intensify premenstrual mood states (Morse and Dennerstein 1988). In our review, four recently published, relevant studies were found in addition to some dissertations.

In one study, four women with prospectively confirmed elevations in premenstrual symptoms were treated with a package that included anger and anxiety management as well as the targeting of negative cognitions (Slade 1989). After an eight-session program, posttreatment premenstrual negative affect measured by the Menstrual Distress Questionnaire (Moos 1968) was significantly reduced compared with baseline levels. Since no control group was used and treatment components were multiple, no causative statements can be made.

Corney and colleagues (1990) offered individually tailored behavior therapy in their study of progesterone, psychotherapy, and pill placebo. Twenty-nine women with a prospectively confirmed diagnosis were given cognitive-behavior psychotherapeutic treatment based on their particular problem areas. The number of individual sessions varied according to the woman's needs and may have included anything from anger management to stress inoculation training. Neither active treatment was found to be superior to placebo as measured in total symptom score on the General Health Questionnaire (Goldberg 1972). The behavior treatment, however, showed a significant advantage in anger management, which was maintained at the 6-month follow-up.

A preliminary, uncontrolled study by Morse and colleagues (1989) of both relaxation and rational-emotive therapy (a form of cognitive therapy) produced positive results in six women with prospectively confirmed symptoms. Women were receiving hormone therapy and participated in 10 weekly group rational-emotive therapy and relaxation sessions, after which all treatments, including hormones, were discontinued. Follow-up assessments at 5 and 11 weeks and at 1 year confirmed significant reductions in symptom clusters, such as concentration and negative affect, reported on the Menstrual Distress Questionnaire (Moos 1968).

This same research group (Morse et al. 1991) conducted a later study comparing hormone therapy (dydrogesterone), coping skill training, and relaxation training in 54 women with prospectively confirmed PMS. Subjects were randomly assigned to groups receiving 1) dydrogesterone (20 mg daily); 2) 10 weekly 90-minute group sessions emphasizing cognitive restructuring, problem-solving, and assertiveness training; or 3) audiotaped relaxation instruction for home practice. Subjects receiving training in coping skills demonstrated significant symptom reductions after 1 month, as measured by the Menstrual Distress Questionnaire (Moos 1968) and the Beck Depression Inventory (Beck et al. 1979). Although the other treatment groups showed initial improvement, only the group receiving training in coping skills maintained these gains at 3 months and showed improvement in concentration. The superiority of cognitive therapy, however, is probably due to the fact that these subjects were engaged in lengthier, more intensive, therapist-assisted treatment, in contrast to how relaxation therapy was administered.

Among dissertations in which cognitive-behavior therapy was compared with control conditions, results were mixed. In a study by Weiss (1988), members of both cognitive-behavior therapy groups and support groups reported decreases in premenstrual depression and anger (as compared with control subjects on a waiting list). At assessments conducted during the luteal phase at 1 and 3 months after treatment, however, only the subjects receiving five sessions of cognitive-behavior therapy showed a significant decrease in negative cognitions, self-blame, and avoidance. Cognitive-behavior therapy may therefore have an additional and differential effect by reducing dysfunctional or negative thoughts.

Byers (1987) examined the effects of 12 group sessions and found the addition of cognitive therapy techniques to be superior to PMS education alone and to assessment control conditions in decreasing dysfunctional attitudes and premenstrual depression. Target symptoms were measured with the Beck Depression Inventory (Beck et al. 1979) and the Dysfunctional Attitudes Survey (Weissman and Beck 1978). In contrast, four individual sessions of cognitive restructuring (Margolis 1985) or cognitive therapy for depression (Leonard 1985) had no significant impact on symptoms when compared with control conditions. These two findings may suggest that the use of an isolated technique (restructuring) is less effective than comprehensive cognitive-behavior therapy, or that very brief interventions (i.e., four sessions) are less likely to produce measurable results.

Relaxation Training

Relaxation training and its variants have been suggested as a method for managing the intensity of premenstrual symptoms such as negative affect, autonomic arousal, and physical discomfort. Coyne (1983) found that women in general exhibited increased muscle tension premenstrually as compared with the follicular phase and that increases in muscle tension in response to a stressful image were greater during the luteal phase. Although these subjects did not have PMS, increased sympathetic arousal was seen as a possible cause of premenstrual symptoms, making relaxation therapy a viable treatment. Deep-muscle relaxation has been shown to be effective in the treatment of spasmodic dysmenorrhea (Chesney and Tasto 1975; Quillen and Denney 1982) and, when paired with relevant cues, may reduce physical feelings of premenstrual heaviness and pelvic pain (Quillen and Denney 1982).

The usefulness of relaxation training in the treatment of premenstrual symptoms is not yet clear, because half of the studies on the subject have evaluated relaxation training as a component of a multifaceted treatment program and not in isolation. The earlier study by Morse and colleagues (1989) combined relaxation and rational-emotive therapy, and although subjects improved after treatment, the relative contribution of relaxation therapy alone could not be evaluated. Reed (1986) included relaxation training as a component in a stress management program and contrasted it with therapist-assisted group therapy and peer-led support. Treatments ran for eight sessions, and all were judged successful on the basis of significant premenstrual decreases in daily symptom ratings. Because the study lacked a no-treatment control group and combined relaxation training with other techniques, however, it is impossible to judge which active treatment components produced positive results. In a dissertation by Weiss (1988), relaxation was also included as part of a cognitive-behavior package. Treatments consisted of five weekly 2-hour group sessions. In this treatment study, cognitive-behavior therapy (with relaxation) was judged to be superior to support group and waiting-list control conditions in reducing maladaptive coping and intensity of negative events. DeWitt (1981) used relaxation training as part of an eight-session physiological treatment package for menstrual and premenstrual distress, but found no posttreatment differences between relaxation training ($n = 4$) and a no-treatment control group ($n = 6$). The small size of the sample in this study, however, could have contributed to the failure to detect modest treatment effects.

Two published studies and one in the dissertation literature did evaluate relaxation training as a single treatment for PMS. The results of a controlled study by Goodale and colleagues (1990) lend support to the relaxation response as an effective aid in reducing both physical and emotional premenstrual symptoms. Diagnoses were prospectively confirmed in 46 women randomly assigned to one of three groups: one that charted symptoms daily, one that read leisure material in addition to charting, and one that practiced relaxation twice a day in addition to charting. Relaxation was practiced at home twice a day with the use of a 7-minute audiotape. Subjects in the relaxation group demonstrated greater reduction in physical and emotional symptoms than the women in the two control groups, as measured by daily ratings and scores on the Premenstrual Assessment Form (Halbreich and Endicott 1982). This effect was particularly pronounced in those women who had higher initial severity scores. Morse and colleagues (1991) did not obtain such impressive results in their comparison of relaxation training, coping skills, and hormone therapy. Initial rapid gains in the relaxation group were not maintained throughout the study, but the research design did not provide an adequate test of the efficacy of relaxation training against cognitive-behavior forms of therapy. Subjects in the cognitive-behavior intervention group received 10 weekly 90-minute sessions led by a therapist; in contrast, subjects in the relaxation group were given an audiotape of an exercise to practice at home. Because guided instruction in proper relaxation technique and consistent practice are often necessary to derive benefits from relaxation training, the negative results reported may only reflect the fact that this training was inadequately administered.

All four studies in which a cognitive or behavior treatment package that included relaxation was used reported improvement of symptoms in subjects, and the usefulness of relaxation alone has been demonstrated in two of the three studies in which this treatment was examined in isolation. Relaxation training appears to be a useful addition to a behavior treatment package for premenstrual symptoms. In addition, its usefulness as a sole treatment for premenstrual changes has also received some support.

Biofeedback

No published studies, and only one dissertation, on the use of biofeedback in subjects with prospectively confirmed PMS were found. Konandreas (1990) administered 12 sessions of combined biofeedback and relaxation to subjects with PMS. The overall mood and well-being of these subjects were significantly improved over those of a control group, as measured by the Profile of Mood States (McNair et al. 1971) but not the Menstrual Distress Questionnaire (Moos 1968). Further studies are necessary before biofeedback can be considered a treatment option, particularly because in this case it was combined with another treatment.

Dietary Changes

A modified diet is one of the most popular treatments recommended for PMS. Although not, strictly speaking, a "psychosocial treatment," dietary modifications do constitute behavioral changes and therefore are included in this review.

Premenstrual lethargy, fatigue, irritability, distractibility, and cravings are considered by some to be due to altered glucose tolerance during the luteal phase (Abraham 1980). Although there appears to be no evidence of altered glucose metabolism during the premenstruum (Denicoff et al. 1990; Spellacy et al. 1990), the results of a study in which nutrient intake was investigated in women with PMS and in control subjects suggest that carbohydrate intake increases premenstrually and may influence mood during the luteal phase (Wurtman et al. 1989). Survey studies have found an association between severe premenstrual symptoms and the consumption of foods and beverages that are high in sugar content (Rossignol and Bonnlander 1991), but such correlational data do not provide evidence that one factor causes the other. In another study, a low-fat, high-carbohydrate diet significantly reduced breast swelling and tenderness in 21 women with long histories of severe premenstrual breast symptoms (Boyd et al. 1988). The existing published studies that report on the use of dietary management in women with carefully diagnosed PMS are either uncontrolled

(Abraham and Rumley 1987; Pearlstein et al. 1992) or combine dietary changes with other treatment components (Pearlstein et al. 1992). Caffeine consumption has also been associated with premenstrual mood and physical changes in survey studies (Rossignol 1985; Rossignol et al. 1989), but no controlled investigation has examined the effect of a reduction in the intake of caffeine.

Although results of some uncontrolled studies suggest that dietary changes such as reduced intake of refined sugar could help to alleviate some symptoms of PMS, no controlled study has examined the isolated effect of dietary modification on premenstrual complaints. An improved diet may be beneficial to general health and well-being, but without a known nutritional etiological factor in PMS, it would appear doubtful that dietary management alone produces lasting symptom changes, at least in severe cases.

Exercise

Exercise is also commonly cited as a treatment for PMS, although no published study has clearly demonstrated its effectiveness as a sole intervention. Timonen and Procope (1971) surveyed 748 female university students and found premenstrual and menstrual complaints to be less common among those who practiced sports. Prior and Vigna (1987) evaluated the effects of exercise on premenstrual symptoms in sedentary women and in runners. Increased exercise was found to be associated with improvements in fluid and breast-related symptoms as well as in premenstrual dysphoria up to 6 months after the beginning of an exercise program, based on daily reports of symptoms. No significant changes in symptoms in control subjects were observed.

Two studies have been undertaken with subjects diagnosed with PMS. Dewitt (1981) included exercise as part of a treatment package for women with self-diagnosed PMS, but posttreatment changes in the symptoms of these women were not found to be significantly different from those of control subjects. Lemon (1991) evaluated the isolated effect of aerobic training in a study of 32 women with prospectively confirmed PMS. Women were randomly assigned to either a high-intensity aerobic training group or a low-intensity control group for 10 weeks. Although the high-intensity group showed greater reductions, both groups demonstrated improvements in comparison with a baseline. Additional controlled studies are needed to clarify whether exercise can help to alleviate physiological and psychological symptoms of PMS.

Conclusions

The somatic treatment studies discussed here represented 31 specific PMS treatments. Frequently, treatments were administered premenstrually and were aimed at relief only of luteal phase symptoms. When administered in a cyclic fashion, treatments such as alprazolam, bromocriptine, buspirone, light therapy, metolazone, naltrexone, and spironolactone were superior to placebo for relief of at least some premenstrual symptoms. The studies of alprazolam are of particular interest, because this is a drug with a high potential for the development of dependence and dose escalation, neither of which were observed in the studies discussed here. Further, alprazolam appeared to provide relief from the full syndrome.

The continuous use of ovulation suppressors was a prominent treatment form in the studies reviewed here. Ovulation suppression achieved through the use of danazol, estradiol, buserelin, and oophorectomy have been shown to effectively halt cyclic fluctuations in reproductive hormone levels, concomitantly decreasing or abolishing severe premenstrual symptoms.

Continuous pharmacologic treatment at doses considered subtherapeutic for disorders such as depression and anxiety have been shown to be efficacious in controlling premenstrual symptoms. One treatment that seems to be effective in a low dose is clomipramine, normally used in the treatment of depression. When used for premenstrual complaints, a low dose of clomipramine is superior to placebo. As might be expected, irritability, and not dysphoria, is the symptom most improved by clomipramine. Other continuous, low-dose treatments that seem to be effective are clonidine, doxycycline, fluoxetine, and propranolol. Fluoxetine seems to be effective in the usual doses recommended for the treatment of depression.

Psychosocial therapies that have thus far been subjected to at least one controlled study with PMS subjects are cognitive-behavior techniques, relaxation training, support groups, and exercise. Although study results are mixed, cognitive-behavior approaches (that encompass a number of techniques such as restructuring, thought-stopping, and anger management) appear to be promising in the treatment of some premenstrual symptoms. Relaxation training, particularly when used in combination with other treatments such as cognitive-behavior therapy, appears to ameliorate physical and sometimes emotional symptoms. At least two studies have examined relaxation training in isolation and have reported positive results.

In the one controlled study that examined its isolated effects, exercise did produce symptom improvement, but the nearly equivalent gains made by control subjects engaging in low-intensity exercise make us question whether this may have been a placebo response. Another possible explanation is that the adoption of a routine of improved self-care, such as one including exercise, and not the type or intensity of activity, may have positive effects on women whose self-esteem and sense of personal control is compromised during the luteal phase.

It is difficult to determine from the studies reviewed here how the support group experience can bring about significant changes in PMS symptoms, because this treatment was often confounded with the inclusion of psychotherapeutic techniques that can themselves promote behavioral change. Therefore, the relative impact of empathic listening and support alone has yet to be adequately evaluated. Psychotherapy coupled with pharmacotherapy also needs evaluation. Finally, dietary modifications (which include reduced intake of refined sugar and caffeine) have not been subjected to controlled trials to clarify the possible relationship between food intake and premenstrual symptomatology.

Although much work remains to be done, clinicians appear to have at their disposal a limited number of pharmacological and psychosocial treatment approaches that may help to control some premenstrual symptoms. In each instance, the risks must be weighed against the benefits of treatment.

References

Abraham GE: Premenstrual tension. Current Problems in Obstetrics and Gynecology 3:3–39, 1980

Abraham G: Nutrition and the premenstrual tension syndrome. J Appl Nutr 36:103–124, 1984

Abraham GE, Hargrove JT: Effect of vitamin B6 on premenstrual symptomatology in women with premenstrual tension syndromes: a double blind crossover study. Infertility 3:155–165, 1980

Abraham GE, Rumley RE: Role of nutrition in managing the premenstrual syndrome. J Reprod Med 32:405–422, 1987

American Psychiatric Association: Diagnostic and Statistical Manual of Mental Disorders, 3rd Edition, Revised. Washington, DC, American Psychiatric Association, 1987

Andersch B, Hahn L: Bromocriptine and premenstrual tension: a clinical and hormonal study. Pharmatherapeutica 3:107–113, 1982

Andersch B, Hahn L: Progesterone treatment of premenstrual tension— a double-blind study. J Psychosom Res 29:489–493, 1985

Andersen AN, Larsen JF, Steenstrup OR, et al: Effect of bromocriptine on the premenstrual syndrome: a double-blind clinical trial. Br J Obstet Gynaecol 84:370–374, 1977

Asberg M, Perris C, Schalling D, et al: The CPRS: development and applications of a psychiatric rating scale. Acta Psychiatr Scand Suppl 271:1–69, 1978

Bancroft J, Boyle H, Warner P, et al: The use of an LHRH agonist, buserelin, in the long-term management of premenstrual syndromes. Clin Endocrinol 27:171–182, 1987

Barr W: Pyridoxine supplements in the premenstrual syndrome. Practitioner 228:425–427, 1984

Beck AT, Rush AJ, Shaw ES, et al: Cognitive Therapy of Depression. New York, Guilford, 1979

Benedek-Jaszmann LJ, Sturtevant H: Premenstrual tension and functional infertility: etiology and treatment. Lancet 1:1095–1098, 1976

Boyd NF, Shannon P, Kriukov, et al: Effect of a low-fat high-carbohydrate diet on symptoms of cyclical mastopathy. Lancet 1:128–132, 1988

Brush MSG: Abnormal essential fatty acid levels in plasma in women with PMS. Am J Obstet Gynecol 150:363–364, 1984

Buss AH, Durkee A: An inventory for assessing different kinds of hostility. J Consult Clin Psychol 21:343–349, 1957

Byers SB: A comparison of the efficacy of education alone or in combination with cognitive therapy in the treatment of premenstrual syndrome. Dissertation Abstracts International 48:3674, 1987

Callender K, McGregor M, Kirk P, et al: A double-blind trial of evening primrose oil in the premenstrual syndrome: nervous symptom subgroup. Human Psychopharmacology Clinical and Experimental 3:57–61, 1988

Campbell A, Converse PE, Rodgers WL: The Quality of American Life: Perceptions, Evaluations, and Satisfactions. New York, Russell Sage, 1976

Carroll BJ, Feinberg M, Smouse PE, et al: The Carroll Rating Scale for Depression, I: development, reliability and validation. Br J Psychiatry 138:194–200, 1981

Casper RF, Hearn MT: The effect of hysterectomy and bilateral oophorectomy in women with severe premenstrual syndrome. Am J Obstet Gynecol 162:105–109, 1990

Casson P, Hahn PM, Van Vugt DA, et al: Lasting response to ovariectomy in severe intractable premenstrual syndrome. Am J Obstet Gynecol 162:99–105, 1990

Chakmakjian ZH, Higgins CE, Abraham GE: The effect of a nutritional supplement, Optivite for Women, on premenstrual tension syndromes, II: effect on symptomatology, using a double blind cross-over design. Journal of Applied Nutrition 37:12–17, 1985

Chesney MA, Tasto DL: The effectiveness of behavior modification with spasmodic and congestive dysmenorrhea. Behav Res Ther 13:245–253, 1975

Chuong C, Coulam C, Bergstralh E, et al: Clinical trial of naltrexone in premenstrual syndrome. Obstet Gynecol 72:332–336, 1988

Corney RH, Stanton R, Newell R, et al: Comparison of progesterone, placebo and behavioral psychotherapy in the treatment of premenstrual syndrome. Journal of Psychosomatic Obstetrics and Gynaecology 11:211–220, 1990

Coyne C: Muscle tension and its relation to symptoms in the premenstruum. Res Nurs Health 6:199–205, 1983

Denicoff KD, Hoban MC, Grover GN, et al: Glucose tolerance testing in women with premenstrual syndrome. Am J Psychiatry 147:477–480, 1990

Dennerstein L, Spencer-Gardner C, Gotts G, et al: Progesterone and the premenstrual syndrome: a double-blind crossover trial. Br Med J 290:1617–1621, 1985

Dennerstein L, Morse C, Gotts G, et al: Treatment of premenstrual syndrome: a double-blind trial of dydrogesterone. J Affect Disord 11:199–205, 1986

DeWitt PH: Comparison of group training procedures for coping with menstrual distress. Dissertation Abstracts International 42:2049, 1981

Endicott J, Spitzer RL, Fleiss JL, et al: The Global Assessment Scale: a procedure for measuring overall severity of psychiatric disturbance. Arch Gen Psychiatry 33:766–771, 1976

Endicott J, Nee J, Cohen J, et al: Premenstrual changes: patterns and correlates of daily ratings. J Affect Disord 10:127–135, 1986

Eriksson E, Lisjo P, Sundblad C, et al: Effect of clomipramine on premenstrual syndrome. Acta Psychiatr Scand 81:87–88, 1990

Evans DR, Burns JE, Robinson WE, et al: The Quality of Life Questionnaire: a multidimensional measure. Am J Community Psychol 13:305–310, 1985

Fortin JN, Wittoker ED, Falz F: A psychosomatic approach to the premenstrual tension syndrome: a preliminary report. Can Med Assoc J 79:978–981, 1958

Frank RT: The hormonal basis of premenstrual tension. Archives of Neurology and Psychiatry 26:1053–1057, 1931

Freeman E, Rickels K, Sondheimer S, et al: Ineffectiveness of progesterone suppository treatment for premenstrual syndrome. JAMA 264:349–353, 1990

Ghose K, Coppen A: Bromocriptine and premenstrual syndrome: controlled study. BMJ 1:147–148, 1977

Giannini AJ, Sullivan B, Sarachene J, et al: Clonidine in the treatment of premenstrual syndrome: a subgroup study. J Clin Psychiatry 49:62–63, 1988

Gilmore DH, Hawthorn RJ, Hart DM: Danol for premenstrual syndrome: a preliminary report of a placebo-controlled double-blind study. J Int Med Res 13:129–130, 1985

Goldberg DP: The Detection of Psychiatric Illness by Questionnaire. London, Oxford University Press, 1972

Goodale IL, Domar AD, Benson H: Alleviation of premenstrual syndrome with the relaxation response. Obstet Gynecol 75:649–655, 1990

Graham JJ, Harding PE, Wise PH, et al: Prolactin suppression in the treatment of premenstrual syndrome. Med J Aust 2:18–20, 1978

Gunston KD: Premenstrual syndrome in Cape Town, II: a double-blind placebo-controlled study of the efficacy of mefenamic acid. S Afr Med J 70:159–160, 1986

Hagen I, Nesheim B, Tuntland T: No effect of vitamin B-6 against premenstrual tension: a controlled clinical study. Acta Obstet Gynecol Scand 64:667–670, 1985

Halbreich U, Endicott J: Classification of premenstrual syndromes, in Behavior and the Menstrual Cycle. Edited by Friedman RC. New York, Marcel Dekker, 1982, pp 243–265

Hamilton M: A rating scale for depression. J Neurol Neurosurg Psychiatry 23:56–62, 1960

Hammarbäck S, Bäckström T: Induced anovulation as treatment of premenstrual tension syndrome: a double-blind crossover study with GnRH-agonist versus placebo. Acta Obstet Gynecol Scand 67:159–166, 1988

Harrison WM, Endicott J, Rabkin JG, et al: Treatment of premenstrual dysphoric changes: clinical outcome and methodological implications. Psychopharmacol Bull 20:118–122, 1984

Harrison WM, Endicott J, Rabkin JG, et al: Treatment of premenstrual dysphoria with alprazolam and placebo. Psychopharmacol Bull 23:150–153, 1987

Harrison WM, Endicott J, Nee J: Treatment of premenstrual depression with nortriptyline: a pilot study. J Clin Psychiatry 50:136–139, 1989

Harrison WM, Endicott J, Nee J: Treatment of premenstrual dysphoria with alprazolam: a controlled study. Arch Gen Psychiatry 47:270–275, 1990

Hartmann L: Presidential address: reflections on humane values and biopsychosocial integration. Am J Psychiatry 149:1135–1141, 1992

Haskett RF, Abplanalp JM: Premenstrual Tension Syndrome: diagnostic criteria and selection of research subjects. Psychiatry Res 9:125–138, 1983

Hoffman JJ: A double-blind crossover clinical trial of an OTC diuretic in the treatment of premenstrual tension and weight gain. Current Therapeutic Research 26:575–580, 1979

Jakubowicz D, Godard E, Dewhurst J: The treatment of premenstrual tension with mefenamic acid: analysis of prostaglandin concentrations. Br J Obstet Gynaecol 91:78–84, 1984

Jordheim O: The premenstrual syndrome. Acta Obstet Gynecol Scand 51:77–80, 1972

Kendall KE, Schnurr PP: The effects of vitamin B6 supplementation on premenstrual symptoms. Obstet Gynecol 70:145–149, 1987

Kerr G, Day J, Munday M, et al: Dydrogesterone in the treatment of the premenstrual syndrome. Practitioner 224:852–855, 1980

Khoo SK, Munro C, Battistutta D: Evening primrose oil and treatment of premenstrual syndrome. Med J Aust 153:189–192, 1990

Konandreas GK: The effect of biofeedback and relaxation on premenstrual syndrome. Dissertation Abstracts International 51:433, 1990

Kullander S, Svanberg L: Bromocriptine treatment of the premenstrual syndrome. Acta Obstet Gynecol Scand 58:375–378, 1979

Lemon D: The effects of aerobic training on women who suffer from premenstrual syndrome. Dissertation Abstracts International 52:563, 1991

Leonard SR: The treatment validity of identifying and treating depression and behavior change symptom clusters in women complaining of the premenstrual syndrome. Dissertation Abstracts International 46:4019, 1985

London RS, Murphy L, Kitlowski KE, et al: Efficacy of alpha-tocopherol in the treatment of the premenstrual syndrome. J Reprod Med 32:400–404, 1987

Mackay C, Cox T, Burrows G, et al: An inventory for the measurement of self-reported stress and arousal. British Journal of Social and Clinical Psychology 17:282–284, 1978

Maddocks S, Hahn P, Moller F, et al: A double-blind placebo-controlled trial of progesterone vaginal suppositories in the treatment of premenstrual syndrome. Am J Obstet Gynecol 154:573–581, 1986

Magos L, Brincat M, Studd JW: Treatment of the premenstrual syndrome by subcutaneous estradiol implants and cyclical oral norethisterone: placebo controlled study. BMJ 292:1629–1633, 1986

Malmgren R, Collins A, Nilsson C: Platelet serotonin uptake and effects of vitamin B-6 treatment in premenstrual tension. Neuropsychobiology 18:83–88, 1987

Margolis A: The use of a cognitive restructuring intervention in the treatment of premenstrual syndrome: a controlled study. Dissertation Abstracts International 47:381, 1985

Mattsson B, von Schoultz B: A comparison between lithium, placebo, and a diuretic in premenstrual tension. Acta Psychiatr Scand 255 (suppl):75–84, 1974

McNair DM, Lorr M, Droppleman LF: EDITs Manual for the Profile of Mood States. San Diego, CA, Educational and Industrial Testing Service, 1971

Mira M, McNeil D, Fraser I, et al: Mefenamic acid in the treatment of premenstrual syndrome. Obstet Gynecol 68:395–398, 1986

Moos RH: The development of a menstrual distress questionnaire. Psychosom Med 30:853–867, 1968

Morse CA, Dennerstein L: Cognitive therapy for premenstrual syndrome, in Functional Disorders of the Menstrual Cycle. Edited by Brush MG, Goudsmit EM. New York, Wiley, 1988, pp 177–190

Morse CA, Bernard ME, Dennerstein L: The effects of rational-emotive therapy and relaxation training on premenstrual syndrome: a preliminary study. Journal of Rational-Emotive and Cognitive-Behavior Therapy 7:98–110, 1989

Morse CA, Dennerstein L, Farrell E, et al: A comparison of hormone therapy, coping skills training and relaxation for the relief of premenstrual syndrome. J Behav Med 14:469–489, 1991

Muse K, Cetel N, Futterman L, et al: The premenstrual syndrome: effects of "medical ovariectomy." N Engl J Med 311:1345–1349, 1984

Nikolai TF, Mulligan GM, Gribble RK, et al: Thyroid function and treatment in premenstrual syndrome. J Clin Endocrinol Metab 70:1108–1113, 1990

O'Brien PMS, Craven D, Selby C, et al: Treatment of premenstrual syndrome by spironolactone. Br J Obstet Gynaecol 86:142–147, 1979

Overall JE, Gorham DR: The Brief Psychiatric Rating Scale. Psychol Rep 10:799–812, 1962

Parry B, Rosenthal N, Tamarkin L, et al: Treatment of a patient with seasonal premenstrual syndrome. Am J Psychiatry 144:762–766, 1987

Parry BL, Berga SL, Mostofi N, et al: Morning versus evening bright light treatment of late luteal phase dysphoric disorder. Am J Psychiatry 146:1215–1217, 1989

Parry BL, Rosenthal NE, James SP, et al: Atenolol in premenstrual syndrome: a test of the melatonin hypothesis. Psychiatry Res 37:131–138, 1991

Pearlstein TB, Rivera-Tovar A, Frank E, et al: Nonmedical management of late luteal phase dysphoric disorder: a preliminary report. Journal of Psychotherapy Practice and Research 1:49–55, 1992

Prior JC, Vigna Y: Conditioning exercise and premenstrual symptoms. J Reprod Med 32:423–428, 1987

Quillen MA, Denney DR: Self-control of dysmenorrheic symptoms through pain management training. J Behav Ther Exp Psychiatry 13:123–130, 1982

Rausch JL, Janowsky DS, Golshan S, et al: Atenolol treatment of late luteal phase dysphoric disorder. J Affect Disorder 15:141–147, 1988

Reed RA: Premenstrual syndrome: the comparative efficacy of three group therapy interventions. Dissertation Abstracts International 47:4312, 1986

Rees L: The premenstrual tension syndrome and its treatment. BMJ 1:1014–1016, 1953

Reid RL: Premenstrual syndrome, in Current Problems in Obstetrics and Gynecology. Edited by Leventhal JM, Hoffman JJ, Keith LG, et al. Chicago, IL, Year Book Medical, 1985, pp 1–57

Richter M, Haltvick R, Shapiro S: Progesterone treatment of premenstrual syndrome. Current Therapeutic Research 36:840–850, 1984

Rickels K, Freeman E, Sondheimer S: Buspirone in treatment of premenstrual syndrome (letter). Lancet 1:777, 1989

Rickels K, Freeman E, Sondheimer S, et al: Fluoxetine in the treatment of premenstrual syndrome. Current Therapeutic Research 48:161–166, 1990

Rossignal AM: Caffeine-containing beverages and premenstrual syndrome in young women. Am J Public Health 75:1335–1337, 1985

Rossignal AM, Bonnlander H: Prevalence and severity of the premenstrual syndrome: effects of food and beverages that are sweet or high in sugar content. J Reprod Med 36:131–136, 1991

Rossignal AM, Zhang J, Chen Y, et al: Tea and premenstrual syndrome in the People's Republic of China. Am J Public Health 79:67–69, 1989

Sampson G: Premenstrual syndrome: a double-blind controlled trial of progesterone and placebo. Br J Psychiatry 135:209–215, 1979

Sampson GA, Heathcote PR, Wordsworth J, et al: Premenstrual syndrome: a double-blind cross-over study of treatment with dydrogesterone and placebo. Br J Psychiatry 153:232–235, 1988

Sarno AP, Miller EJ, Lundblad EG: Premenstrual syndrome: beneficial effects of periodic, low-dose danazol. Obstet Gynecol 70:33–36, 1987

Singer K, Cheng R, Schou M: A controlled evaluation of lithium in the premenstrual tension syndrome. Br J Psychiatry 124:50–51, 1974

Slade P: Psychological therapy for premenstrual emotional symptoms. Behavioral Psychotherapy 17:135–150, 1989

Smith S, Rinehart JS, Ruddock VE, et al: Treatment of premenstrual syndrome with alprazolam: results of a double-blind, placebo-controlled, randomized crossover clinical trial. Obstet Gynecol 70:37–43, 1987

Spielberger CD, Gorsush RL, Lushene RE: State Trait Anxiety Inventory (STAI) Manual. Palo Alto, CA, Consulting Psychologists Press, 1970

Spellacy WN, Ellingson AB, Keith G, et al: Plasma glucose and insulin levels during the menstrual cycles of normal women and premenstrual syndrome patients. J Reprod Med 35:508–511, 1990

Steiner M, Haskett RF, Carroll B: Premenstrual tension syndrome: the development of research diagnostic criteria and new rating scales. Acta Psychiatrica Academica 62:117–190, 1980a

Steiner M, Haskett R, Osmun J, et al: Treatment of premenstrual tension with lithium carbonate. Acta Psychiatr Scand 61:96–102, 1980b

Steiner M, Haskett RF, Osmun JN, et al: The treatment of severe premenstrual dysphoria with bromocriptine. Journal of Psychosomatic Obstetrics and Gynaecology 2:223–227, 1983

Stephenson MJ, Milner R, Lamont J, et al: Treatment of premenstrual syndrome with oil of evening primrose: a randomized controlled trial. Proceedings of the 16th Annual Meeting of the North American Primary Care Research Group, Ottawa, Ontario, Canada, 1988

Stewart A: Clinical and biochemical effects of nutritional supplementation on the premenstrual syndrome. J Reprod Med 32:435–441, 1987

Stone AB, Pearlstein T, Brown W: Fluoxetine in the treatment of late luteal phase dysphoric disorder. J Clin Psychiatry 152:290–293, 1991

Sundblad C, Modigh K, Andersch B, et al: Clomipramine effectively reduces premenstrual irritability and dysphoria: a placebo controlled study. Acta Psychiatr Scand 85:39–47, 1992

Thys-Jacobs S, Ceccarelli S, Bierman A, et al: Calcium supplementation in premenstrual syndrome: a randomized crossover trial. J Gen Intern Med 4:183–189, 1989

Timonen S, Procope BJ: Premenstrual syndrome and physical exercise. Acta Obstet Gynecol Scand 50:331–337, 1971

Toth A, Lesser M, Naus G, et al: Effect of doxycycline on premenstrual syndrome: a double-blind randomized clinical trial. J Int Med Res 16:270–279, 1988 van der Meer YG, Benedek-Jaszmann LJ, van Loenen AC: Effect of high-dose progesterone on the premenstrual syndrome: a double-blind cross-over trial. Journal of Psychosomatic Obstetrics and Gynaecology 2-4:220-222, 1983

Vellacott ID, Shroff NE, Pearce MY, et al: A double-blind, placebo-controlled evaluation of spironolactone in the premenstrual syndrome. Curr Med Res Opin 10:450–456, 1987

Walton J, Youngkin E: The effect of a support group on self-esteem of women with premenstrual syndrome. J Obstet Gynecol Neonatal Nurs 16:174–178, 1987

Watson NR, Savvas M, Studd JWW, et al: Treatment of severe premenstrual syndrome with oestradiol patches and cyclical oral norethisterone. Lancet 2:730–732, 1989

Watts JF, Edwards RL, Butt WR: Treatment of premenstrual syndrome using danazol: preliminary report of a placebo-controlled, double-blind, dose ranging study. J Int Med Res 13:127–128, 1985

Watts JF, Butt WR, Edwards RL: A clinical trial using danazol for the treatment of premenstrual tension. Br J Obstet Gynecol 94:30–34, 1987

Weiss CR: Cognitive behavioral group therapy for the treatment of premenstrual distress. Dissertation Abstracts International 49:2389, 1988

Weissman AN, Beck AT: Dysfunctional Attitudes Scale. Springfield, VA, ERIC Document Reproduction Service, 1978

Werch A, Kane R: Treatment of premenstrual tension with metolazone: a double-blind evaluation of a new diuretic. Current Therapuetic Research 19:5651572, 1976

Williams MJ, Harris R, Dean B: Controlled trial of pyridoxine in the premenstrual syndrome. J Int Med Res 13:174–179, 1985

Wood C, Jakubowicz D: The treatment of premenstrual syndromes with mefenamic acid. Br J Obstet Gynaecol 87:627–630, 1980

Wurtman J, Brzezinski A, Wurtman RJ, et al: Effect of nutrient intake on premenstrual depression. Am J Obstet Gynecol 161:1228–1234, 1989

Ylostalo P, Kauppila A, Poulakka J, et al: Bromocriptine and norethisterone in the treatment of premenstrual syndrome. Obstet Gynecol 59:292–298, 1982

Zuckerman M, Lubin B: Manual for Multiple Affect Adjective Check List. San Diego, CA, Education and Industrial Testing Services, 1965

ꙅ 6 ꙅ

Commentary on the Literature Review

Mary Brown Parlee, Ph.D.

> New data are abundant in our complex and lively field,
> but there is relatively little agreed upon integration of
> the biopsychosocial data. That contributes to a split be-
> tween researchers and clinicians.
>
> Hartmann 1992, p. 1138

During the past 25 years, premenstrual syndrome (PMS) has
become a topic of systematic scientific research. This chapter
focuses on Chapters 1, 3, and 5, which reflect the efforts of the
American Psychiatric Association (APA) Work Group on Late
Luteal Phase Dysphoric Disorder (LLPDD). These chapters provide a clear, comprehensive, and up-to-date review of the biomedical literature.[1] They are the basis for recommendations in
the DSM-IV regarding the status of the diagnosis of LLPDD.

Literature reviews are particularly difficult because detailed
and technically complex research articles have to be synthesized
into relatively simple (or at least relatively short) verbal summaries
and conclusions. To fully appreciate the scope and complexity of
the task with which the APA work group was charged, I attempted
to reverse this process: to begin with the verbal summaries in the
review and go behind them to the data in the original articles. In
doing this, I became convinced of the usefulness of a set of statistical techniques, called meta-analysis, that provides reviewers with a

quantitative basis for arriving at conclusions about a body of research. Meta-analyses have become increasingly widely used in the social sciences over the past 15 years, and their potential usefulness for biomedical research topics is beginning to be recognized. Because they are well suited to some of the purposes of the APA work group's review, I briefly describe them and their potential uses here.

Close consideration of the data in PMS research articles also underscored for me two solid empirical facts that are usually not discussed in this literature in the way I will characterize them. Because I think they are of considerable scientific significance, the main part of my discussion focuses on these facts and on their methodological and conceptual implications.

The Literature Reviewer's Task

If one looks in detail at individual research articles in the PMS literature, it is clear that at each step in the analysis of the data (including the initial choice of self-report instruments), investigators must necessarily have made choices about how to score, combine, and compare the data from individual women. Other choices could equally reasonably be made and often were made by other PMS researchers reporting their results in other articles. Reviewers summarizing data across studies using slightly different instruments and techniques must also in their turn make choices. For example, in some of the PMS treatment studies compiled by the APA work group, ovulation suppression was found to be superior to placebo for relief of some PMS symptoms, whereas in other studies it was not; some symptoms were relieved in some studies, other symptoms in others; sometimes tests of statistical significance just failed to reach the conventional $P < .05$ level, but a trend seems apparent if one looks at the data. How can the reviewer decide which of these disparate investigations provide the most relevant and reliable data on which to base summaries and conclusions about research on the effectiveness of ovulation suppression or other pharmacologic treatments?

In short, if the reviewer wants to rely on data, and especially the best data, to reach and justify a conclusion about a body of research, he or she is confronted with the task of deciding what to do with studies that differ in details both large and small. Is there a procedure for making empirically based decisions about how to combine and weigh individual investigations to arrive at a conclusion about the research topic that best reflects the body of existing data as a whole? Some answers, according to an increasing number of social scientists, may come from a recently codified body of statistical procedures called meta-analysis.

Meta-analysis of PMS Research: The Example of Treatment Studies

The term *meta-analysis* in the sense referred to here was first used by Glass (1976) to refer to a set of statistical techniques for analyzing and integrating the results of a large number of individual research studies on a single topic. *Primary analysis* is analysis of data from a single investigation; *secondary analysis* is a reanalysis of data from a single study, using new techniques to answer different questions; *meta-analysis* is a statistical analysis of the findings of many studies. The data for a meta-analysis can be the means, standard errors, t or F values, χ^2, or even probability levels from a combined group of individual studies.

Because it can be both quantitative and flexible, meta-analysis is believed to offer advantages over traditional narrative reviews or "vote-counting" reviews. (The latter involves simple tallies of significant and nonsignificant studies.) According to one recent monograph, the "quantitative summary of research domains" (Rosenthal 1991, p. 4) that meta-analysis provides

> go[es] beyond the traditional reviews in the degree to which they are more systematic, more explicit, more exhaustive, and more quantitative. Because of these features, meta-analytic reviews are more likely to lead to summary statements of greater thoroughness, greater precision and greater subjectivity or objectivity. (Rosenthal 1991, p. 11)

For example, in an empirical comparison of conclusions drawn from narrative and from meta-analytic reviews of the same research domain, Wolf (1986) reported that a small but significant effect was identified through the use of meta-analyses that was overlooked or discounted in the narrative review.

For the reviewer seeking to arrive at general, data-based conclusions about research on PMS or LLPDD treatment, meta-analysis offers at least three advantages. First, meta-analysis makes it possible to combine the results of many studies to calculate an overall probability that a difference between data from two groups would have been observed by chance (i.e., the difference between the treatment and control conditions). Because a meta-analysis can summarize the combined data from several studies, it is sensitive to results from individual investigations that are nearly but not quite statistically significant, which would be lost if the findings from single studies were simply tallied as either significant or not.

Second, by coding individual investigations in various ways, it is possible for the meta-analyst also to weigh studies according to quality (as defined by the reviewer) and to evaluate quantitatively their relationship to the presence or absence of significant differences between the groups in the combined results. It is also possible to evaluate quantitatively the contribution of different parameters of the studies that may be of interest. For example, it would be possible to determine whether psychological or physical symptoms are more clearly affected by treatments, whether some kinds of treatments are more effective than others, whether some psychological measures are more sensitive to treatment effects than others, and whether large sample studies more reliably show effects than small sample studies.

Third, meta-analytic techniques can be used to provide a quantitative estimate of the size of the effect of an experimental manipulation (or group difference) relative to the estimated variance in the population. For example, we know from research on sex differences in psychology that a statistically significant difference between two groups may be found even when the absolute difference between population means is small—if the sample size is very large. How do we determine whether this statistically significant difference is scientifically or socially significant? By providing a quantitative measure across a group of studies of effect size relative to standard deviations, a meta-analysis can provide more information than a simple significant-difference test, This information may be useful in assessing the scientific (and perhaps clinical and social) significance of the data.

The techniques of meta-analysis thus appear to be a useful complement to traditional methods of literature review.[2] I have outlined their potential application in reviews of PMS treatment research in the hope that others interested in evaluating PMS research on this and other topics will also begin to use these new techniques.[3] If reasonable disagreements persist about any of the research areas reviewed by the APA work group, it might be possible to resolve them on the basis of information provided by meta-analyses.

Solid But Neglected Facts in PMS Research

Despite areas of potential disagreement, however, my reading of the APA work group's review and the literature on which it is based highlighted two solid empirical facts in the PMS literature, the existence and nature of which all serious researchers agree upon. Given their status as unchallenged facts in a field in which many questions remain unanswered, I believe their scientific implications merit further research.

Fact 1

At present *there is only one method by which researchers identify women with "true" PMS, or with "prospectively confirmed" LLPDD.* Women are given self-rating, self-report, or visual analog scales to complete during one or more menstrual cycles, and scientific criteria are applied to the ratings to identify those women who have PMS or LLPDD.[4] It is a solid, undeniable, empirical fact that, given our present state of knowledge, there is no other way, apart from such psychological data, to know for research purposes whether or not a woman "has" PMS/LLPDD.[5]

Although PMS and LLPDD have rich and multiple meanings in everyday language and in clinical experience, in research they are (are only, until otherwise demonstrated) a particular pattern of responses made by a woman on self-rating scales. In the language of experimental research, this means that the operational definition of PMS as a particular pattern of self-reports has not been externally validated. It has not been shown to be associated with other data, measured independently, from either the biological or the behavioral realm. When an operationally defined construct is "method dependent," as is presently the case in PMS research, assumptions underlying the interpretation of the data produced by using this method require especially careful scrutiny and testing.

From a scientific point of view, therefore, the self-rating data are central to the PMS research enterprise. They would also, by extension, be central to any clinical decisions relying on systematic empirical research for their rationale. For these reasons, it is important to consider evidence for the validity, both internal and external, of self-rating data in PMS research.

Internal validity of self-rating data. Different kinds of data can be obtained from self-rating scales (some are categorical data, some ordinal, some ratio), and each has well-known psychometric properties that determine the kinds of statistical analyses that can be performed on them without violating their underlying assumptions. Some statistics (both descriptive and hypothesis testing) are more "robust" than others and are still interpretable when some of their underlying assumptions are violated in different ways. Statisticians have worked out fairly well, both empirically and theoretically, which procedures can tolerate what kinds of violations, and this specialized area of statistical expertise is clearly relevant for PMS research.

In practice, however, the psychometric properties of self-rating scales are often disregarded in the scientific literature on PMS. Women's responses on questionnaire scales are usually analyzed as though they were ratio data (as though they were, for example, measures of weight or height). They are added together, across women and often across symptoms and moods, as if there were equal intervals between the scale items and an absolute reference point for all women and for clusters of symptoms and emotions. The data are treated as though, for example, the difference between "no bloating" and "mild bloating" has the same meaning as the difference between "mildly impaired concentration" and "severely impaired concentration," or as if one woman's meaning when she checks "extremely angry" is the same meaning as another's.

Although researchers often indicate their awareness of some of these assumptions—when they refer to "subjective" ratings, for example—their research methods only infrequently address this problem directly, and the rating data are analyzed as though the numbers were objective measures.[6] For example, only one of the articles (Hammarbäck and Bäckström, 1988) reviewed in Chapter 5 explicitly raises the issue of the psychometric properties of self-rating data and uses methods of statistical analysis appropriate to such data. The work of Bäckström and his students is promising as a sign that PMS researchers are beginning to address some hitherto neglected methodological issues.

Self-rating data, the central focus in PMS research, are not simple, objective measures of internal psychological states (though upon careful analysis and empirical investigation they may turn out to approximate this fairly closely). What we know for certain now is that they are data—check marks on a questionnaire—produced when investigators administer questionnaires to women under certain conditions. These data have particular psychometric properties that require appropriate methods of analysis to preserve the internal validity of PMS research. It is not just the psychometric properties of the data, however, that are important in PMS research. Procedures for establishing their external validity—their scientific meaning, and ultimately their human meaning and clinical significance—are also important.

External validity of self-rating data. Several years ago, there was a debate among scientists about the validity of menstrual distress

questionnaires—about what women's responses on such questionnaires mean or represent (Asso 1983; Parlee 1982). This debate
appears now to have been resolved, with most investigators agree-
ing that prospective self-ratings are the appropriate way in which
to measure cycle-related symptom and mood changes, because interpretation of data from retrospective menstrual distress questionnaires is still subject to dispute (as possibly being more
influenced by cultural beliefs). The methodological resolution,
however, is only a partial solution to the problem of external validity and of the scientific meaning of the prospective data.

What does it mean when a woman checks "very severe" for a
particular symptom or mood on a self-rating scale in a PMS study?
More precisely, how does the scientist know what this check mark
means to the woman? The investigator's interpretation of the data
(check marks) refers to the woman's feelings, thoughts, and ac-
tions, but how does she or he evaluate the validity of this? So-called
face validity (the check mark means what it "says" it means—she is
telling us that she has very severe mood swings) is somewhat helpful but is clearly not acceptable as the sole criterion for validity.

Ambiguity about the meaning of the data is unnecessarily compounded when research reports do not provide specific and clear
information about the actual procedures by which the self-rating
data were obtained by the investigators. For example, the precise
instructions to the subject and her perceptions of the experiment
are rarely reported. Was the woman asked to rate her "mood
swings" during the previous 24 hours? If so, are her ratings affected
by the time of day she completes the questionnaire or by the length
of time since her last meal? Did she believe her responses would
affect her access to treatment for PMS? Procedural details such as
these are known to affect the outcome in some kinds of psychological research. Their role in PMS research remains to be examined
empirically to establish the external validity of data obtained from
self-report questionnaires.

In short, it is an unremarked but undeniable fact that the phenomenon under investigation in PMS research is measured, assessed, and/or defined in only one way: as a pattern of check marks
women make on self-rating scales administered by the investigator.

These data have specific psychonomic properties and are appropriately analyzed only with particular statistical procedures. In addition to the threats to internal validity posed by inappropriate use of statistics, the external validity of self-rating data has not yet been fully established. To begin to do this, researchers will need to empirically investigate details of experimental procedures that are currently left unreported in most journal articles. PMS research will become more rigorous and more definitive only insofar as investigators recognize that obtaining and analyzing psychological data is in many ways as technically difficult and dependent on specialized skills and knowledge as is collection, analysis, and interpretation of biological data.

Fact 2

The second undeniable empirical fact highlighted by the APA work group's review comes from PMS treatment research, where the data clearly show that *the placebo effect is reliable, ubiquitous, and substantial.* It is found even in research in which the subject population has been carefully screened to include only women with "confirmed" or "true" PMS (Watson et al. 1989). The existence and pervasiveness of the placebo effect has often been noted by PMS researchers (e.g., Sampson 1987). It too, however, has been addressed methodologically, as a technical issue, and its implications for the conceptualization of research questions have been neglected.

The most rigorous treatment studies, those screened and included in the APA work group's review, now use placebo-controlled trials of active treatments to assess the treatment's effect. There are very good reasons for using such a research design in treatment trials.[7] This resolution of the "problem" of the placebo effect, however—construing it as a methodological problem to be addressed through changes in research design—again sidesteps the scientifically fundamental question of what the phenomenon means. In addition, it obscures an underlying question about the validity and the scientific meaning of self-rating data in PMS research. What is the meaning of these data, these check marks on questionnaires, which change so demonstrably when placebo treatment is given?

In a body of research literature in which significant effects are relatively difficult to obtain consistently and the central phenomenon (PMS, assessed solely by self-ratings) has been only weakly validated in research, why have investigators not identified the placebo effect as a substantive phenomenon worthy of further research in its own right? Why have they not empirically determined the psychometric properties and external validity of their self-rating data? Prompted by two undeniably solid empirical facts in the PMS literature, such research clearly would expand our scientific knowledge base about PMS. To do so, however, investigators would need to identify explicitly and test empirically some assumptions about PMS that they have been tacitly endorsing in their research.

Implications of Facts 1 and 2:
Investigate PMS as an Illness, Not a Disease

Some anthropologists distinguish between *illness* or *sickness* and *disease* in a way that may be helpful in clarifying certain assumptions and issues in PMS research (Young 1982). A disease in this sense is the physically observable biological abnormality associated with a medical condition. Illness or sickness is the outcome of sociocultural and psychological processes by which a person comes to label certain features of her or his experience as *symptoms,* seeks medical advice, and receives a diagnosis. A psychological feeling or behavior that is labeled as a symptom may well have an independently observable, biologically specifiable disease process as a cause. The individual's history and social-psychological milieu, however, necessarily play a part in the interpretation and labeling (by the individual and the people in her or his immediate social environment) of the psychological feeling or behavior as a symptom requiring consultation with a medical professional rather than as, say, a manifestation of disordered spiritual life requiring consultation with a religious leader. The notion of illness thus entails, as the notion of disease does not, consideration of the social, cultural, and psychological processes through which persons experience bodily states as having subjective and social meanings. (Kleinman and Good's (1985) introduction to *Culture and Depression* discusses these issues in some detail, with clinical examples.)

In this anthropological sense, then, a person might have the disease of cancer but would not have the illness of cancer, with all its cultural resonances and subjective ramifications (Sontag 1978), unless or until the diagnosis were made by a physician. A disease process such as physical wasting or starvation might be regarded as an illness (e.g., anorexia nervosa) in one culture and a sign of spiritual refinement in another (Bynum 1987). At the psychological level, which is the level tapped by self-rating instruments in PMS research, it seems reasonable to hypothesize (and to test the hypothesis) that the cultural interpretation of a particular bodily state influences an individual's subjective, embodied experiences of a physical condition. In the examples here, the experiences might be characterized globally as "sickness" or as "saintliness".[8]

Research evidence clearly shows that PMS is an illness. Many women notice aspects of their experience that cause them distress and that they think of as symptoms: they respond to researchers' calls for volunteers with PMS and they spontaneously seek a physician's advice and help. When they are diagnosed as having PMS and are treated by a physician, often they get better. These women experience genuine suffering and are genuinely helped by their physicians. PMS is a "real" illness in every reasonable sense, and as such it seems to be an appropriate focus for concern, regardless of whether a biological disease process is involved.

Further research is needed to clarify whether PMS is a disease. It might, of course, be both an illness and a disease. The APA work group has concluded that, to date, a biological marker for the condition has not been identified. A great deal of research has been, and undoubtedly will continue to be, done to discover such a marker, research guided by what is aptly named a "disease model" of PMS. The undeniably solid fact of a placebo effect, however, suggests that a fruitful direction for further research would be to investigate PMS conceptualized as an illness as well.

Empirical research guided by an illness model of PMS might be carried out by using the conceptual frameworks and methodological techniques developed by social psychiatrists and social scientists to study other illness processes (Tishelman et al. 1991). For example, under what circumstances does a woman identify an experience of anger as a symptom? (Laws [1983] provides an analysis of this.) How, that is, in what terms, does she present her distress in the clinician's office? What responses does she get? How are family interactions changed, if at all, by a diagnosis of PMS? Research conducted to answer questions like these would broaden our scientific knowledge base about PMS. It is not incompatible with, and is not an alternative to, research on PMS conceptualized according to a disease model.

Broader Contexts of PMS Research

Directions for further research, such as research on the internal and external validity of the self-rating scales that operationally define PMS, investigation of the substantive meaning of the placebo effect, and the use of new statistical techniques such as meta-analysis, would provide a more complete scientific picture of PMS than is presently available. Scientific research on any topic is always incomplete in important respects: this is usually what stimulates scientific fields to continue to change and develop. In the case of PMS research, it is an empirical question, to which we will all know the answer in 5 or 10 years, whether investigators will take seriously the implications of what I have called Facts 1 and 2 (and what others have discussed under different rubrics) and will use a broader range of methods and conceptualizations than are currently being employed by the many able investigators in this field. Alternatively, will PMS research continue along present lines, with questions framed according to the assumptions of a disease model only, validity problems with self-report data remaining unaddressed, and quantitative methods for literature reviews being underutilized?

Cognitive rigidity within a scientific or professional community, like cognitive rigidity within an individual, manifests itself by lack of flexibility in the face of new data and lack of resourcefulness in developing new solutions to previously neglected or ignored facts. Scientific research on PMS has become very much more rigorous during the past 25 years. It has done this by adopting methodological canons of the natural sciences, pursuing investigations in which psychological data are conceptualized as objective phenomena and PMS is presumed to be a direct result of a disease process. This work will and, I think, should continue.

Reviews and summaries of this work, however, when they are as carefully done as they have been by the APA Work Group on LLPDD, direct our attention to the actual data behind the summaries. In so doing, they uncover additional methodological and theoretical issues and facts whose genuine scientific significance has been overlooked. For a scientific community to take these seriously and investigate them with appropriate methodologies, it will have to be flexible: to be open to reexamining basic assumptions and to be able to adopt new methods and conceptual frameworks as required by thoughtful and careful consideration of all the data.

In the case of PMS research in particular, this means giving more careful and informed consideration to the psychological data that literally define the phenomenon for research purposes. It means finding new and better ways to determine what women who participate in PMS research are doing and experiencing in their own terms, what they are "saying" with their responses on the self-rating scales, and what they say when "asked" by other methods borrowed from the social sciences, anthropology, and the clinician's office (Good and Good 1981). Closer attention to (i.e., more rigorous standards for addressing) methodological and conceptual issues surrounding the psychological data in PMS research seems likely to result in a greater diversity of research paradigms.

If, in 5 or 10 years' time, the APA Work Group on LLPDD were to be again charged with reviewing the literature, I hope they will find that it is more diverse methodologically and more rigorous conceptually. If so, our scientific understanding of PMS will be more comprehensive and empirically grounded, and therefore will be of greater clinical relevance. If this is the case, I think it will

be because the APA work group's current review has been so clear
and comprehensive that it has illuminated both the strengths and
limitations of existing research and thereby points to promising
directions for the future.[9]

Notes

1. The APA work group's members, with Dr. Judith Gold as Chair,
   have done an outstanding job of identifying pertinent issues
   and assembling and evaluating an extremely complex research
   literature on a controversial topic. As an experimental psychologist who has done research on the menstrual cycle for more
   than 20 years, I understand very well the amount of sheer hard
   work that went into the effort of bringing so much and such
   varied data into some kind of meaningful coherence. The APA
   work group's thoughtful review contributes to our clearer understanding of this field and provides a useful framework for
   further research.
2. Literature reviews using meta-analyses, research about the
   technique itself, and textbooks and computer programs for
   using meta-analysis have all appeared with rapidly increasing
   frequency during the past decade (see references in Glass et al.
   1981; Rosenthal 1991; Wolf 1986). Meta-analysis has even been
   featured in general-interest publications (Stipp 1992), which is
   no doubt a sign that it is, as Rosenthal (1991) has suggested, a
   "revolution in the making" (p. 10) in the behavioral and biomedical sciences.

   I admit to initial skepticism over the enthusiasm that meta-
   analysis has been generating among psychologists. A badly designed study or a poorly formulated research question cannot
   be reconceptualized by combining its results with data from
   other investigations, and there is surely no substitute for the
   kind of critical thought that structures a good narrative review.
   These and other misgivings and objections, however, have
   been explicitly addressed by proponents of meta-analysis (as a
   complement to traditional review methods), and I have come

to see the usefulness of the techniques for certain research questions and problems.

3. In reading research articles on PMS treatments with an eye to performing meta-analyses on the data they reported, it became apparent that conventions regarding the publication of empirical findings differ from journal to journal. In research reports in psychological journals, psychologists are required to be very detailed about the self-rating instruments used (exactly what the items and response options are and empirical data on their validity and reliability, or references to articles in which this information is fully reported). Failure of journal editors to require this detailed reporting is usually a sign of a lower-quality journal. Furthermore, in reporting data from two groups or on two conditions, high-quality psychological journals require the reporting of means and standard deviations of the data from both groups or conditions, as well as the *t* or *F* values (for parametric tests) and the associated *P* values. To an experimental psychologist, these data are as crucial for interpreting the research as I imagine are detailed descriptions of how gonadal hormone levels were measured to a biomedically trained scientist. The frequent absence or lack of stringent reporting standards for behavioral data in the PMS treatment studies, in fact, stands in marked contrast to the detail and thoroughness with which parameters of the menstrual cycle itself are measured and reported.

4. In a careful analysis of existing data sets, Hurt and colleagues (1992) demonstrated that the specific criteria applied to prospective ratings to define PMS can affect researchers' estimates of the incidence and prevalence of the illness. In the case of an individual woman, the particular criterion applied might determine whether the provisional diagnosis of LLPDD is prospectively confirmed. Regardless of variations among the criteria used, however, all are applied to the same kind of data: self-reports obtained from pencil-and-paper instruments completed by the woman on a daily basis. The data of Hurt and colleagues (1992) also suggest the potential usefulness of an analysis of the relationships between the specific items and re-

sponse options that make up particular self-report instruments and incidence and prevalence estimates.

5. In a review of the literature on PMS published in *Psychological Bulletin* more than 20 years ago (Parlee 1973), I concluded that

> studies of the premenstrual syndrome have not as yet established the existence of a class of behaviors and moods, *measureable in more than one way* [original emphasis], which can be shown in a longitudinal study to fluctuate throughout the course of the menstrual cycle. (p. 463)

In this respect, despite considerable progress in research (including demonstration of cycle-related fluctuations in behaviors not clinically significant), the scientific status of premenstrual syndrome remains unchanged. I also emphasized in that review that "this is not to say that such a set of behaviors does not exist—many women spontaneously attest that they *do* [emphasis added]" (Parlee 1973, p. 463), and this too remains unchanged.

6. The term *objective* is used here in the specific philosophical sense that an object can be known objectively when it can be completely understood from the outside, from the observer's perspective.

7. Although these criteria for methodologically adequate treatment research may seem obvious today, it is important to remember that they were not always so, and that a great deal of scientific work over nearly two decades has gone into making them widely accepted. My intention here is to try to build on this progress, identifying some additional criteria for methodological adequacy in LLPDD research that may come to seem equally obvious in the future.

8. One advantage of using this anthropological framework for conceptualizing research about PMS is that it avoids the dichotomies of body versus mind, "real" versus "all in the head," and nature versus culture. These are unnecessary conceptual traps that sometimes sidetrack or even polarize scientific discussions rather than move them toward more constructive research questions.

9. Although it is an empirical question whether a disease model will continue to predominate exclusively in PMS research during the next decade, it is tempting to speculate on some of the alternatives. What might we say, for example, if in 5 or 10 years PMS research is largely unchanged, having addressed none of the issues I raise here and that many others have raised many times before me and in other contexts?

Scientific rigidity in the face of the intractable facts and unresolved problems of the sort I discuss here seems likely to perpetuate problems of validity and gaps in knowledge and to forestall the development of a body of cumulatively coherent, empirically based knowledge about PMS. Such rigidity in a scientific research community, due to institution-based incentives and reward structures that incline investigators to cling to models that unduly restrict the scope of inquiry and to disregard facts incompatible with tacit, widely shared assumptions, might suggest that processes other than scientific ones are operating to influence the research enterprise (Latour 1987). Disagreements in PMS research and discussions of LLPDD have sometimes involved claims by one or more of the parties that politics is or should not be influencing science (Asso 1983; Schacht 1985; Spitzer 1985). Given the present state of the field—the facts, the gaps, and the availability of additional methods and conceptual frameworks—continued exclusive predominance of a disease model in PMS research during the next 5 or 10 years would be presumptive evidence of scientific rigidity. It would also lend force to the argument of those who believe that sometimes doing science is engaging in politics by other means (Smith 1990). A version of this argument has in fact been made with specific reference to the development of and changes in the diagnostic categories of the DSM (Brown 1990; Caplan 1991). My hope is that scientific flexibility, rather than rigidity, will prevail in PMS research during the next decade. The data will tell.

References

Asso D: The Real Menstrual Cycle. Chichester, England, Wiley, 1983

Brown P: The name game: toward a sociology of diagnosis. The Journal of Mind and Behavior 11:385–406, 1990

Bynum C: Holy Feast and Holy Fast: The Religious Significance of Food to Medieval Women. Berkeley, University of California Press, 1987

Caplan PJ: How do they decide who is normal? the bizarre, but true tale of the DSM process. Can J Psychol 32:162–170, 1991

Glass G: Primary, secondary, and meta-analysis of research. Educational Researcher 5:3–8, 1976

Glass GV, McGaw B, Smith ML: Meta-analysis in Social Research. Beverly Hills, CA, Sage, 1981

Good BJ, Good MJD: The meaning of symptoms: a cultural hemeneutic model for clinical practice, in The Relevance of Social Science for Medicine. Edited by Eisenberg L, Kleinman A. Boston, MA, Reidel, 1981, pp 165–196

Hammarbäck S, Bäckström T: Induced anovulation as treatment of premenstrual tension syndrome: a double-blind crossover study with GnRH-agonist versus placebo. Acta Obstet Gynecol Scand 64:393–397, 1988

Hartmann L: Presidential address: reflections on humane values and biopsychosocial integration. Am J Psychiatry 149:1135–1141, 1992

Hurt SW, Schnurr PP, Severino SK, et al: Late luteal phase dysphoric disorder in 670 women. Am J Psychiatry 149:525–530, 1992

Kleinman A, Good B (eds): Culture and Depression: Studies in Anthropology and Cross-Cultural Psychiatry of Affect and Disorder. Berkeley, University of California Press, 1985

Latour B: Science in Action. Cambridge, MA, Harvard University Press, 1987

Laws S: The sexual politics of premenstrual tension. Women's Studies International Forum 6:19–31, 1983

Parlee MB: Premenstrual syndrome. Psychol Bull 80:454–465, 1973

Parlee MB: The psychology of the menstrual cycle: biological and psychological perspectives, in Behavior and the Menstrual Cycle. Edited by Friedman RC. New York, Marcel Dekker, 1982, pp 77–99

Rosenthal R: Meta-Analytic Procedures for Social Research, revised edition. Newbury Park, CA, Sage, 1991

Sampson GA: Premenstrual syndrome: characterization, therapies, and the law, in Premenstrual Syndrome: Ethical and Legal Implications in a Biomedical Perspective. Edited by Ginsburg BE, Carter BF. New York, Plenum, 1987, pp 301–316

Schacht TE: DSM-III and the politics of truth. Am Psychol 40:513–521, 1985

Smith DE: The Conceptual Practices of Power. Boston, MA, Northeastern University Press, 1990

Sontag S: Illness as Metaphor. New York, Farrar, Straus & Giroux, 1978

Spitzer RL: DSM-III and the politics-science dichotomy syndrome: a response to Thomas E. Schacht's "DSM-III and the politics of truth." Am Psychol 40:522–526, 1985

Stipp D: Medical experts slow to adopt new remedies. Wall Street Journal, July 8, 1992, pp B1, B4

Tishelman C, Taube A, Sachs L: Self-reported symptom distress in cancer patients: reflections of disease, illness or sickness? Soc Sci Med 11:1229–1240, 1991

Watson NR, Studd JWW, Savvas M, et al: Treatment of severe premenstrual syndrome with oestradiol patches and cyclical oral norethisterone. Lancet 2:730–732, 1989

Wolf FM: Meta-analysis: Quantitative Methods for Research Synthesis (Quantitative Applications in the Social Sciences series, Vol 59). Beverly Hills, CA, Sage, 1986

Young A: The anthropology of sickness and the anthropology of illness. Annual Review of Anthropology 11:257–285, 1982

II

Sociocultural Issues

❧ 7 ☙

Historical Perspective of Premenstrual Syndrome

Judith H. Gold, M.D., F.R.C.P.C.

> To assume, as we all do, that biochemical processes un-
> derlie mental activity and behaviour does not imply that
> they are the causal agents but rather constitute mediat-
> ing mechanisms. They are influenced by the informa-
> tion inputs we receive from our body and environment
> and by the subjective meaning of that information for
> us. It is that meaning which largely determines what we
> think, feel and do.
>
> Lipowski 1989, p. 252

Historically, by the 7th century, literature reported that there were twice as many cases of mental disorder among women than men; by the 19th century, most of the patients in mental institutions were women from all social classes and circumstances (Showalter 1985). In her book *The Female Malady,* Showalter (1985) observed further that

> the prevailing view among Victorian psychiatrists was that . . .
> women were more vulnerable to insanity than men because the
> instability of their reproductive systems interfered with their sex-
> ual, emotional, and rational control. . . . This connection be-
> tween the female reproductive and nervous systems led to the

condition nineteenth-century physicians called "reflex insanity
in women." (pp. 55–56)

She continued by quoting from physicians of that time who
related menses to insanity and who concurred that menstrual
blood predisposed to mental illness. They developed special
bloodletting techniques and special diets designed to regulate
menstruation and gave advice to mothers on methods that might
delay menarche in their daughters.

Physicians in the late 19th century concentrated on the effects
of exercise and education on women's health and menstrual functioning. Henry Maudsley "felt that the 'extraordinary expenditure
of vital energy' made through the establishment of menstruation
during the critical years of puberty (and after) left 'little vitality to
spare' for other functions" (Showalter 1985, p. 125). In 1879, Na-
than Allen wrote about the disastrous effects of education on the
mental functioning and physiology of young women who were not
in good physical condition because of their lack of vigorous exercise. He felt that mentally a woman could not withstand the rigors
of learning unless she was exercising (Allen 1879). Both of these
men were writing and teaching in a milieu where great attention
was paid to female "hysteria," "anorexia," and "neurasthenia." All
were viewed as causally related to sexuality, masturbation, and
menstruation:

> Although the discourses describing ostensible causes of hysteria
> changed over time, from physiology to moral failings to the haz-
> ards of modern society, a woman's sanity was consistently tied to
> her reproductive system and her role in society. (Rodin 1992,
> p. 51)

In fact, empirical knowledge consisted of anecdotal clinical reports influenced by social conventions. Formal studies meeting
current standards did not exist. Novelists, playwrights, and artists
exploited the subject of female mental illness, although a few—
such as John Stuart Mill—wrote about the deleterious effects on
women of their social circumstances. Formal exploration of the

possible relationship of the menstrual cycle with mental illness began only in the 20th century and is attributed to R. T. Frank, who in 1931 described a premenstrual tension syndrome in 15 subjects. Like his predecessors, he prescribed bloodletting as a successful treatment that enabled the excretion of sex hormones. Late in that decade, S. L. Israel (1938) was the first to suggest the existence of a progesterone deficiency. By 1953, Greene and Dalton had coined the term *premenstrual syndrome* (PMS [Speroff 1988]). In research following in the footsteps of Frank, Israel, and Dalton, PMS was studied from the perspective of a medical model focusing on hormones and physiology. Such research is reviewed in Chapters 1, 3, 4, and 5.

As Severino and Moline (1989) described in their historical review of PMS, there was another perspective following from the pioneering work of Freud:

> [Freud] viewed disturbances of menstruation as a model for determining the effect of a physical disturbance on ego functioning. He believed that a weak ego was the decisive factor in the genesis of a neurosis. He also believed that a physical illness could weaken the ego and produce a neurosis. Thus a disturbance of menstruation could theoretically result in a condition in which a woman's instincts were too strong for the enfeebled ego to cope with them. (Severino and Moline 1989, p. 12)

Other psychoanalysts (see review by Severino 1991) also theorized about premenstrual symptoms being linked to anger about being female, ambivalence about pregnancy, and conflicts about sexual preference. Freud and his followers, although introducing the concept of mind influencing biology, remained true to the biomedical model with its focus on disease:

> The dominant model of disease today is biomedical, with molecular biology its basic scientific discipline. It assumes disease to be fully accounted for by deviations from the norm of measurable biological (somatic) variables. It leaves no room within its framework for the social, psychological, and behavioral dimensions of illness. (Engel 1977, pp. 129–130)

Others with sociological, cultural, and historical orientations have contributed to the behavioral perspective of menstruation. This behavioral perspective and its elaboration by those assessing the sociocultural determinants of behavior are addressed in Chapters 8 and 9. This perspective views PMS and LLPDD as "a recreation of tacit cultural knowledge about the effect of the reproductive system on women's behavior" (Rodin 1992, p. 50).

The Phenomenology of Late Luteal Phase Dysphoric Disorder

The phenomenological description of late luteal phase dysphoric disorder (LLPDD) must be understood in the context of PMS. Brush and Goudsmit (1988) quote Dalton's definition of PMS as "the recurrence of symptoms on or after ovulation, increasing during the premenstruum and subsiding during menstruation, with complete absence of symptoms from end of menstruation to ovulation" (p. 3). Katherina Dalton's work led to the popular view in society that PMS is a "bona fide" condition of women.

However, there is no consistent definition of PMS. It has been used as a pejorative term in regard to women's behavior and competency, with the result that the perception of the general public is that women can be unreliably moody at "that time of the month" (Chrisler and Levy 1990). Thus, women present themselves in physicians' offices and at PMS clinics stating that they have PMS and want treatment. The lack of a consistent definition has made the interpretation of research data from such populations difficult and replication or comparison of studies almost impossible.

Many health researchers with an interest in PMS because of the affective symptoms experienced by women met in 1983 at a conference sponsored by the National Institute of Mental Health (NIMH). At that meeting, more specific guidelines were set for determining how much change there must be in symptom severity, where in the menstrual cycle change should occur, and how the change should be documented in order for a woman to be diagnosed as having PMS. It was decided that documentation by prospective daily symptom ratings was required and that these ratings must show "mean symptom intensity changes of at least 30% in the premenstrual period (6 days before menses) compared with the intermenstrual period (days 5–10 of the cycle)" (Parry et al. 1985, p. 88).

In 1987, the DSM-III-R (American Psychiatric Association 1987) Task Force of the American Psychiatric Association more specifically defined a dysphoric disorder associated with the menstrual cycle that resulted in social and occupational impairment, as distinct from the general physical and less severe mood symptoms of PMS. This mental disorder was called *late luteal phase dysphoric disorder.* However, since it was decided that further research is required to validate its existence, LLPDD was placed in a research appendix to DSM-III-R. Its definition can be found in Table 7–1.

Only a few years later, an agreement was made between the United States and the World Health Organization to coordinate the contents and coding of the 10th edition of the *International Classification of Diseases* (ICD-10 [World Health Organization 1992]) and DSM. A task force was appointed to develop DSM-IV. The older term *premenstrual tension,* coined by Frank (1931), is included in the ICD nomenclature under "Diseases of the Genitourinary system (N00–N99): N94, Pain and other conditions associated with female genital organs and the menstrual cycle."

The DSM-IV Task Force was to reexamine DSM-III-R and make any revisions or additions found to be scientifically necessary. A work group was formed within this task force to study the diagnosis of LLPDD and to determine whether sufficient data existed in research studies to justify its classification as a mental disorder or, if not, whether it should remain in the appendix of DSM-IV to be studied further. The basic issues to be examined were the validity and clinical usefulness of this proposed new disorder as described in the appendix of DSM-III-R; that is, was there a clinically significant mental disorder associated with the menstrual cycle, and could it be distinguished from other mental disorders?

The work group began with a review of the literature on

LLPDD. Because LLPDD had entered the nomenclature only in the appendix to DSM-III-R in 1987, published studies were limited. Relevant PMS literature was, therefore, also reviewed. The litera-

---

Table 7–1. Diagnostic criteria for late luteal phase dysphoric disorder

A. In most menstrual cycles during the past year, symptoms in B occurred during the last week of the luteal phase and remitted within a few days after the onset of the follicular phase. In menstruating females, these phases correspond to the week before, and a few days after, the onset of menses. (In nonmenstruating females who have had a hysterectomy, the timing of luteal and follicular phases may require measurement of circulating reproductive hormones.)

B. At least five of the following symptoms have been present for most of the time during each symptomatic late luteal phase, at least one of the symptoms being 1, 2, 3, or 4:

   1. Marked affective lability, e.g., feeling suddenly sad, tearful, irritable, or angry

   2. Persistent and marked anger or irritability

   3. Marked anxiety, tension, feelings of being "keyed up" or "on edge"

   4. Marked depressed mood, feelings of hopelessness, or self-deprecating thoughts

   5. Decreased interest in usual activities, e.g., work, friends, hobbies

   6. Easy fatigability or marked lack of energy

   7. Subjective sense of difficulty in concentrating

   8. Marked change in appetite, overeating, or specific food cravings

   9. Hypersomnia or insomnia

   10. Other physical symptoms, such as breast tenderness or swelling, headaches, joint or muscle pain, a sensation of bloating, weight gain

C. The disturbance seriously interferes with work or with usual social activities or relationships with others.

D. The disturbance is not merely an exacerbation of the symptoms of another disorder, such as major depression, panic disorder, dysthymia, or a personality disorder (although it may be superimposed on any of these disorders).

E. Criteria A, B, C, and D are confirmed by prospective daily self-ratings during at least two symptomatic cycles. (The diagnosis may be made provisionally prior to this confirmation.)

Source. Reprinted from *Diagnostic and Statistical Manual of Mental Disorders,* 3rd Edition, Revised. Washington, DC, American Psychiatric Association, 1987, p. 369. Used with permission. Copyright 1987 American Psychiatric Association.

ture reviewed used data bases from Medline, *Psychological Abstracts, Index Medicus,* the Biological Retrieval Service, and Medlars obtained on a monthly basis until the end of 1991. Over 400 articles were reviewed (Gold et al., in press).

Essential portions of the work group's literature review can be found in Chapters 1, 3, 5, and 8. The literature review, although comprehensive and current, is limited by the facts that there were still (through 1991) few published studies of LLPDD and that methodological problems still existed in PMS and LLPDD studies that precluded a meaningful synthesis of the findings. The methodological problems are described in detail in Chapters 2 and 6. These problems include variability in the number of days included, differences in the number of days after the onset of menses, how the symptoms were recorded and elicited, how severe they were, and whether any of these were even stated in the published articles. Many studies did not use control groups or used very small samples with few women. Furthermore, the PMS studies mostly did not use prospective daily ratings, resulting in heterogeneous samples of women.

To address the methodological problem of how to measure symptom change, the work group reanalyzed existing data on women from five different sites who sought help for premenstrual symptoms. This reanalysis estimated the prevalence of the LLPDD symptoms and overall diagnosis in these treatment-seeking women as a function of four different statistical methods for determining symptom change. The analysis showed that the prevalence of LLPDD varied depending on which scoring method was used (Severino et al., in press). Based on this data reanalysis, the phenomenology of LLPDD was changed (Table 7–2). The name LLPDD was also changed to premenstrual dysphoric disorder (PMDD).

Future Directions

LLPDD has been described phenomenologically as a cyclic mood disorder of women who experience a cluster of symptoms

Table 7–2.   Diagnostic criteria for premenstrual dysphoric disorder (PMDD)

A. In most menstrual cycles during the past year, symptoms in C occurred during the last week of the luteal phase and began to remit within a few days after the onset of the follicular phase, and are absent in the week after menses. In menstruating females, the luteal phase corresponds to the period between ovulations and the onset of menses and the follicular phase begins with menses. (In nonmenstruating females, e.g., those who have had a hysterectomy, the timing of luteal and follicular phases may require measurement of circulating reproductive hormones.)

B. The disturbance markedly interferes with work and school or with usual social activities and relationships with others (e.g., avoidance of social activities or decreased productivity and efficiency at home and at work).

C. At least five of the following symptoms have been present for most of the time during each symptomatic late luteal phase, at least one of the symptoms being 1, 2, 3, or 4:

1. Markedly depressed mood, feelings of hopelessness, or self-deprecating thoughts

2. Marked anxiety, tension, feelings of being "keyed up" or "on edge"

3. Marked affective lability (e.g., feeling suddenly sad or tearful or increased sensitivity to rejection)

4. Persistent and marked anger or irritability or increased interpersonal conflicts

5. Decreased interest in usual activities (e.g., work, school, friends, hobbies)

6. Subjective sense of difficulty in concentrating

7. Lethargy, easy fatigability, or marked lack of energy

8. Marked change in appetite, overeating, or specific food cravings

9. Hypersomnia or insomnia

10. Subjective sense of being overwhelmed or out of control

11. Other physical symptoms, such as breast tenderness or swelling, headaches, joint or muscle pain, a sensation of bloating, weight gain

D. The disturbance is not merely an exacerbation of the symptoms of another disorder, such as major depressive disorder, panic disorder, dysthymic disorder, or a personality disorder (although it may be superimposed on any of these conditions).

E. Criteria A, B, C, and D must be confirmed by prospective daily ratings during at least two symptomatic cycles. (The diagnosis may be made provisionally prior to this confirmation.)

Source.   Reprinted from *DSM-IV Draft Criteria.* Washington, DC, American Psychiatric Association, 1993. Used with permission. Copyright 1993 American Psychiatric Association.

specific to the late luteal phase of the menstrual cycle. Operationally, LLPDD is a particular pattern of responses made by a woman on a self-rating scale that is method dependent for diagnosis. The external validity of self-rating data has not been fully established. Women view symptoms differently and so differ in their scoring of severity. For some women, premenstrual symptoms are perceived as a normal physiological reality, not as an "illness" or as incapacitating (Facchinetti et al. 1992). A woman's attitude toward and expectations about menstruation can influence how she rates the severity of the symptoms or even acknowledges their existence. The issues of comorbidity (Christensen et al. 1992) and of social and cultural influences (Raja et al. 1992), discussed in other chapters, also influence symptom ratings. It is important to a full understanding of premenstrual symptoms and to research methodology that an optimal symptom scoring procedure be determined. A measure of functional impairment also must be established.

An epidemiological study of PMS or LLPDD has not been conducted to date based on prospective daily ratings. A 1990 study of university women who were unaware of the purpose of the study and who gave over 90 days of daily ratings gave a point prevalence of 4.6% using LLPDD criteria (Rivera-Tovar and Frank 1990). A retrospective study during the Epidemiological Catchment Area study at the Duke University site, in Durham, North Carolina, using seven questions from the LLPDD criteria, noted an overall prevalence of 6.8% (Stout and Steege, ASPOG Annual Meeting, New York, 1990). A general population study by Haskett and colleagues (R. F. Haskett, A. DeLongis, R. C. Kessler, unpublished data, May 1987) showed a prevalence of 3.4% for PMS. Others have reported that 20%–40% of women report premenstrual symptoms, with about 5% saying these have a significant impact on their lives (American College of Obstetricians and Gynecologists 1989). A review of the literature does not demonstrate that these symptoms are related to psychoses, despite earlier historical attempts to do so (Gold et al., in press; Severino and Yonkers 1993).

The etiology of LLPDD remains unknown. Additionally, the course of premenstrual symptoms over the years of a woman's life has not been delineated. It is not known whether they remain the same, grow worse or better with age, or vary from one symptomatic month to another in type or severity. Clinical impression is that those seeking treatment for PMS are usually in their 30s, although symptoms can begin at any time after menarche and usually remit with menopause. There are no data available for LLPDD.

Studies of familial risk factors for LLPDD are lacking. A Finnish study reported that 70% of daughters with mothers with "premenstrual tension" also had symptoms, compared with only 37% of daughters of unaffected mothers (Kantero and Widholm 1971). One study (Dalton et al. 1987 [N = 15 monozygous twins, 16 dizygous twins, and 77 sibling control subjects]) reported that symptoms of PMS are likely to occur in both monozygotic twins or not at all. Concordance rates were significantly higher in monozygotic twins (93%) than in dizygotic twins (44%) or in sibling control subjects (31%). The difference between dizygotic twins and sibling control subjects was not significant. A retrospective self-report study of 827 same-sex twins (zygosity assigned by an algorithm) reported that familial resemblance for premenstrual symptoms was due solely to genetic factors 35.1% of the time (Kendler et al. 1992).

Conclusions

The new criteria for PMDD emphasize the dysphoric nature of the disorder. They require severe impairment and minimize the physical complaints. This disorder is clearly one of mood but is associated with the premenstruum. Some findings from studies of the etiology and treatment of premenstrual symptoms suggest that the mechanism for mood symptoms may be similar to that for other mood disorders. The data are comparable in quantity and quality to those of other conditions currently classified as mental disorders.

PMDD, however, is a disorder occurring only in women. A similar cyclical disorder in men has not been sought and thus could exist. The legal and social implications associated with the stigma of mental illness and attitudes toward women remain to be understood. Furthermore, sociocultural data suggest that PMDD may be a disorder of certain middle-class, "Western" women. Thus, the relative strength of the data is confounded by some important variables that are not found in other mood disorders.

Efforts to find an independent measure (biological or behavioral) to validate PMDD must continue, but prevalence studies in the general population are needed above all. Just as studies of schizophrenias and of mood disorders have been multicentered worldwide, so should be studies of PMDD. It is vital that the question of a mental disorder related to menstruation be elucidated at last. The threat of stigmatizing women should not prevent clinicians and researchers from understanding the meaning of the symptoms that women report. Women deserve to have PMDD researched, identified, and treated. They do not deserve to be stigmatized by it, any more than androgen disorders stigmatize men. Research into this disorder is essential, and demonstrating a cyclical disorder, whether affecting both women and men or either, will benefit both.

References

Allen N: The Education of Girls, as Connected With Their Growth and Physical Development. Boston, MA, TW Bicknell, 1879

American College of Obstetricians and Gynecologists: Premenstrual syndrome. Committee Opinion No 66. Washington, DC, American College of Obstetricians and Gynecologists, 1989

American Psychiatric Association: Diagnostic and Statistical Manual of Mental Disorders, 3rd Edition, Revised. Washington, DC, American Psychiatric Association, 1987

Brush MG, Goudsmit EM: General and social considerations in research on menstrual cycle disorders with particular reference to PMS, in Functional Disorders of the Menstrual Cycle. Edited by Brush MG, Goudsmit EM. Chichester, England, Wiley, 1988, pp 1–13

Chrisler JC, Levy KB: The media construct a monster: a content analysis of PMS articles in the popular press. Women Health 16:89–104, 1990

Christensen AP, Board BJ, Oei TPS: A psychosocial profile of women with premenstrual dysphoria. J Affect Disord 25:251–260, 1992

Dalton K, Dalton M, Guthrie K: Incidence of the premenstrual syndrome in twins. BMJ 295:1027–1028, 1987

Engel GL: The need for a new medical model: a challenge for biomedicine. Science 196:129–135, 1977

Facchinetti F, Romano G, Fava M, et al: Lactate infusion induces panic attacks in patients with premenstrual syndrome. Psychosom Med 54:288–296, 1992

Frank RT: The hormonal basis of premenstrual tension. Arch Neurol Psychiatry 26:1053–1057, 1931

Gold JH, Endicott J, Frank E, et al: Late luteal phase dysphoric disorder: literature review, in DSM-IV Sourcebook, Vol 2. Washington, DC, American Psychiatric Association (in press)

Greene R, Dalton K: The premenstrual syndrome. British Medical Journal 1:1007–1014, 1953

Israel SL: Premenstrual tension. JAMA 110:1721–1723, 1938

Kantero RL, Widholm O: Statistical analysis of the menstrual patterns of 8,000 Finnish girls and their mothers, IV: correlations of menstrual traits between adolescent girls and their mothers. Acta Obstet Gynecol Scand Suppl 14:30–36, 1971

Kendler KS, Silberg JL, Neale MC, et al: Genetic and environmental factors in the aetiology of menstrual, premenstrual and neurotic symptoms: a population-based twin study. Psychol Med 22:85–100, 1992

Lipowski ZJ: Psychiatry: mindless or brainless, both or neither? Can J Psychiatry 34:249–254, 1989

Parry BL, Rosenthal NE, Wehr TA: Research techniques used to study premenstrual syndrome, in Premenstrual Syndrome: Current Findings and Future Directions. Edited by Osofsky HJ, Blumenthal SJ. Washington, DC, American Psychiatric Press, 1985, pp 87–95

Raja SN, Feehan M, Stanton WR, et al: Prevalence and correlates of the premenstrual syndrome in adolescence. J Am Acad Child Adolesc Psychiatry 31:783–789, 1992

Rivera-Tovar AD, Frank E: Late luteal phase dysphoric disorder in young women. Am J Psychiatry 147:1634–1636, 1990

Rodin M: The social construction of premenstrual syndrome. Soc Sci Med 35:49–56, 1992

Severino SK: Menstrual cycle experience, in Female Psychology: An Annotated Psychoanalytic Bibliography. Edited by Schuker E, Levinson NA. Hillside, NJ, Analytic Press, 1991, pp 183–193

Severino SK, Moline ML: Premenstrual Syndrome: A Clinician's Guide. New York, Guilford, 1989

Severino SK, Yonkers K: A review of psychotic symptoms associated with the premenstruum. Psychosomatics 34(4):299–306, 1993

Severino SK, Albernathy T, Frank E, et al: Late luteal phase dysphoric disorder: MacArthur Foundation data reanalysis, in DSM-IV Sourcebook, Vol 4. Washington, DC, American Psychiatric Association (in press)

Showalter E: The Female Malady: Women, Madness and English Culture, 1830–1980. New York, Pantheon, 1985

Speroff L: Historical and social perspectives, in The Premenstrual Syndrome. Edited by Keye WR Jr. Philadelphia, PA, WB Saunders, 1988, pp 3–14

World Health Organization: International Classification of Diseases, 10th Edition. Geneva, World Health Association, 1992

ॐ 8 ॐ

Social, Political, and Legal Considerations

Nada L. Stotland, M.D.,
and Bryna Harwood, B.A.

> Social change alters brain cells. . . . Humane values re-
> quire us, in promoting mental health and fighting men-
> tal illness, to be aware of and care for and treat *whole*
> *people in context* and *over time:* whole biopsychosocial peo-
> ple in context and over time.
>
> Hartmann 1992, p. 1137

This chapter is included not only as one facet of the review of the literature relevant to premenstrual dysphoria, but also to address the considerable controversy within the psychiatric, other mental health, and general communities surrounding menstrually related diagnoses (Caplan 1991). Different views have been expressed by members of the American Psychiatric Association's Task Force on the Diagnostic and Statistical Manual of Mental Disorders, Fourth Edition (DSM-IV) and by members of its Work Group on Late Luteal Phase Dysphoric Disorder (LLPDD). One view was that the process can and should begin with a review of data on the self-reported incidence, severity, and effect of symptoms, psychiatric comorbidity, biological correlates, and response to treatment of women with LLPDD (American Psychiatric Association 1987) or premenstrual syndrome (PMS). Guiding this view was the assumption that diseases exist as objective realities independent of psychological, social, historical, political, and legal contexts, and that these aspects of the problem can be considered after the existence of the diagnostic entity is established. There was an implicit assumption that the failure to include such a "validated" diagnosis would represent a concession to political pressure on the "scientific" process.

Another view held that diagnostic entities are nothing more or less than social constructs formulated to serve psychological, social, political, and legal functions. Diagnoses are imbricated in a cultural context that may cause them, that gives them meaning, and that governs the responses of individuals and institutions to them and their use in society. An illness is whatever people in a particular culture define it to be (Fabrega 1989). What contemporary Western culture calls schizophrenia, people in other times and places have rigorously exorcised as possession by evil spirits, or revered as revelations from beneficent deities.

At this point in time, medical and sociocultural forces are demanding more rigor in the delineation of a new diagnosis or treatment than for one that has proved its clinical and social usefulness over decades (Kutchins and Kirk 1989). This is problematic for the diagnosis of LLPDD, because psychological symptoms associated with the menstrual cycle are difficult to delineate as separate from the influence of cultural expectations and gender roles (Koeske and Koeske 1975). The scientific study of premenstrual symptoms or of the psychological concomitants of other aspects of reproductive issues is, therefore, a double-edged sword for women. The symptoms associated with menstruation, pregnancy, and menopause have not received appropriate attention from the medical and scientific community. Women assert that neither their psychiatrists nor their gynecologists are informed or informative about the usual emotional and behavioral manifestations of these normal developments in the reproductive system, nor about their place in women's lives in our society (Parlee 1980). Rather than offering expert assessment of and advice about women's concerns, physicians may recommend surgery or hormonal treatment or may dismiss complaints as unfounded or inevitable (Hellerstein 1984; Youngs and Reame 1985).

Female reproductive organs have been perceived by the medical profession and by society in general as troublesome and expendable (Scully and Bart 1973). The United States has had the highest rate of hysterectomy in the world. To alleviate other symptoms, physicians artificially supplement or manipulate reproductive hormones. These interventions predate more recent studies linking postmenopausal hormone therapy with a decreased incidence of osteoporosis and heart disease. Gynecologists debate about whether menopause is a deficiency disease or a healthy development that is insufficiently understood. Scientific and clinical attention to hormonal and reproductive events affecting half the human race is long overdue.

At the same time, the "medicalization" of female reproductive events lends itself to a "pathologizing" that also has a long history (Lothstein 1985). Menstruation has been widely referred to in U.S. society as "the curse" (Delaney et al. 1976). "Hysteria" is a well-known and ancient example of the tendency to blame unwelcome behavior and incomprehensible symptoms on female reproductive organs. There has long been evidence of cyclical and noncyclical, but significant, variability in men's psychological states and functions (Hersey 1931). Men's emotional cycles, and associations between male reproductive hormones and socially deleterious behaviors, however, have not been addressed in psychiatric nosology.

Social stigma is not commensurate with actuarial data. For example, automobile insurance for adolescent males is considerably more costly than for people of any other age and gender. There seems to be an association between the surge of male hormones and the risk to people and property, but no "testosterone-related conduct disorder of adolescence" has been proposed. The official labeling of symptoms related to menstruation, pregnancy, and menopause as mental illness threatens to stigmatize women as unstable, unreliable, and inferior.

Few women in, or desirous of, positions of responsibility would choose to mention, much less request help for, reproductivity-related problems. The frequency with which these issues are aired and, especially, acted upon is related to both class and culture (Brooks et al. 1977; Shye and Jaffe 1991). There are many anecdotal reports of absence from work of women in lower-status occupations on grounds of dysmenorrhea. Women in executive and professional positions, and women who work at jobs without sick leave to support families, cannot afford to absent themselves from the workplace for reproductivity-related complaints. In the tenuous positions in which women find themselves in our society at this point in time, the risk of complaints is perceived to be significant. Are professional women stifling a real need for help with symptoms, or are underpaid women expressing their discontent with and noninvolvement in their subordinate positions and their identification with their socially construed frailty?

Katherina Dalton, M.D., of Great Britain, is probably the best-known writer on premenstrual symptoms. An illustrative quote from the preface of her 1969 book (Dalton 1969) expresses ideas that have tremendous currency in both the medical and lay communities on both sides of the Atlantic. The preface was written by Tom E. Dalton, her husband and ghostwriter, and reflects the beliefs of the book's author:

> These findings she has set down in this book so that all who read it may understand the extent to which the cyclical changes in the levels of a woman's hormones are responsible for her unpredictable changes of personality. The reader will begin to realize that there is a biological basis for much that has been written, or said, about the whims and vagaries of women.
>
> The old cliche "It's a woman's privilege to change her mind" calls for an even greater tolerance than before now that it is realized that every woman is at the mercy of the constantly recurring ebb and flow of her hormones. (p. vii)

Dalton repeats these themes in her 1979 book (Dalton 1979), in which she credits PMS for the lack of more disastrous concomitants of the menstrual cycle. She suggests that because women in the premenstrual phase lack the capacity for the clear thinking and careful planning necessary to commit suicide, they are less successful at their attempts (Dalton 1979).

It may be argued that research on menstrually related symptoms is designed to overturn popular misconceptions such as these. Because these ideas derive from cultural beliefs and have achieved wide currency, however, there is also danger that any formalization of PMS as a psychiatric disorder will reify this image of all women. Work based on and citing Dalton continues to appear in the literature (Coughlin 1990; Winter et al. 1991). Dalton's basic reasoning prevails in many ongoing arguments in favor of incorporating the diagnosis into our official nosology. The danger is that establishing that women's purported vagaries are biologically based and causally related to their reproductive hormones absolves women of responsibility for their dangerous moods and behaviors. Such a result would posit and reify the myth of intrinsic female inferiority, unreliability, and incompetence.

A major fallacy (Hurt et al. 1992) in the study of menstrually related changes has been the assumption that the gathering of ever-more precise and varied measures of hormonal relationships and physiological and psychological events will validate those relationships and events as a disease entity. This assumption has led to the basic methodological, sociological, political, legal, and philosophical issues addressed in this chapter.

Anthropological and Historical Perspectives

Menstruation in many so-called primitive societies inspires awe and dread. The menstrual flow, the menstrual condition, and the menstruating woman are seen as polluting. Orthodox Jewish women must avoid not only sexual, but also physical, contact with their husbands during their menstrual periods and immerse themselves after each period in ritual baths to cleanse themselves (Reik 1964). In other societies, women are isolated in "menstrual huts," are forbidden to prepare men's food during menstruation, and are subject to other taboos surrounding menstruation (Stephens 1961). Menstruation necessitates some means to deal with the flow and entails some risk of making a mess. These realities can be burdensome in primitive and technologically developed societies alike. Although the main impact of these burdens might be expected to manifest during menstruation, it is also possible that the anticipated stress would have a negative psychological effect during the premenstruum.

A related gender variable is the preponderance of women in health surveys of illness, days missed from work on grounds of illness, and health service utilization (Verbrugge 1979). Most health surveys are retrospective, and there are few studies examining the relationship between health care utilization and objective pathology. There are several possible explanations for the gender difference in illness behavior. Women may be constitutionally weaker than men, although their longer life spans and other findings mitigate against this. Women's reproductive functions might contribute; for example, the burden of pregnancy and childbirth may damage vital organs. Textbooks of obstetrics and gynecology have tended to espouse the view that female reproductive functions are debilitating and dangerous (Scully and Bart 1973). Although there have been attempts to correct these attitudes in newer texts, the mature cadre of physicians providing reproductive health care to women were educated by these older texts and their authors.

Gender-related functions could also contribute indirectly to poor health; women might have hypertension or back strain secondary to the psychological and physical demands of caring for dependent family members. Some argue that it is women's assumption of dual roles, in the home and in the workplace, that has increased their vulnerability to symptoms. It is women who are at home full-time and who are caring for more than one preschool child, however, who are at highest risk of depressive illness. Women might be socialized to see themselves as sick and to seek health care. Conversely, it has also been argued that men's relative reluctance to obtain medical diagnosis and treatment has a deleterious effect on their own well-being.

The overrepresentation of women as patients could be a cause and/or an effect of menstrually related complaints. The menstrual cycle could make women vulnerable to the onset or exacerbation of medical and psychiatric disorders, or it could itself be so symptomatic for some women as to constitute a disease (Hamilton et al. 1989; Harrison and Endicott 1989; Youngs and Reame 1985). Conversely, women's tendencies to see themselves as ill, complain of symptoms, miss work because of illness, and seek health care could distort their perceptions of cyclical changes into symptoms and illness (Heilbrun and Frank 1989; McEwen 1988; Metcalf et al. 1989).

Women's reproductive functions have been a major factor in the method of scientific exploration of medical questions. The possibility that women subjects might be or might become pregnant has led to their exclusion from studies of many pharmacologic agents and other medical treatments. That most researchers are male may contribute to the tendency to ignore this major limitation on our knowledge of drug safety and possible gender influences on pharmacokinetics, clinical efficacy, and side effects. The same holds true for racial differences. Perhaps potential researchers fear that attempts to identify gender differences would be seen as inegalitarian. The relative lack of female researchers, and the need for them to win research support from traditional sources, also shape the research questions that have been asked. The perception of women as weakened by their reproductive functions, the reality of women's secondary place in society, and the concentration on pathology in medicine lead to research questions focused on negative experiences, reinforcing the circumstances that give rise to them. Research on positive concomitants of the menstrual cycle is rare (Stewart 1989).

The Forensic Arena

Diagnostic labels carry legal implications in most cultures. The history of gender in Western criminal law is interesting. In the 19th century, women were believed to be so naturally angelic as to be incapable of violence. Women who did commit violent crimes were therefore considered not simply bad, but devilish. Links were proposed between crime and psychiatric illness and between psychiatric illness and the menstrual cycle. Women's crimes were blamed on "sensuality" (Chait 1986). During the 20th century, a supposed increase in violent crimes committed by women was attributed to the effects of "women's liberation," although no significant increase occurred. Women make up over 50% of the U.S. population but commit only about 10% of the violent crimes. Arrests of women for murder and manslaughter declined between 1977 and 1983. In general, men are arrested five times as often as women.

The diagnosis of PMS has been introduced in the forensic arena. In two criminal cases in Great Britain in the early 1980s, the women defendants used "premenstrual syndrome" as a defense (Laws 1983, 1990). One woman had threatened to kill a police officer with a knife. She had been sentenced for many crimes in the past and had been undergoing treatment with progesterone injections for a condition that, she argued, caused her to become "a raging animal each month." She was placed on probation with a requirement of medical treatment. The other woman was accused of killing her boyfriend by running him over with her car. PMS was used to reduce the charge from murder to manslaughter under the "diminished capacity" theory. The defendant received a discharge, with the condition that she obtain medical treatment. These cases received a good deal of press in the United States and were soon followed by an attempt to use PMS as a defense in a criminal case in New York. The New York case ended in plea bargaining; the two sides differed as to whether this compromise reflected an acknowledged weakness of the proposed defense (Holtzman 1988).

The possible use of a menstrually related diagnosis as a legal defense embodies the double bind described earlier in this chapter. If some small number of women should be so incapacitated by premenstrual symptoms as to lose control of their behavior, such a plight should be admissible as evidence and should have an impact on the adjudication of their culpability. The implications of headlines linking the menstrual cycle to "raging animals," however, are dire. They reinforce the cultural stereotypes and stigmatization of all women. This real danger necessitates particularly meticulous study and rigorous application of diagnostic criteria. The former is in progress; it is dubious whether the latter can be attained, particularly in courts of law. One lawyer in writing on the subject recommends that, in cases where premenstrual changes may have played a role in a defendant's behavior, her lawyer cite them as organic disease and not as a form of insanity (Chait 1986).

Other Methodologic Problems and Their Implications

The road to a scientific definition of menstrually related symptoms has been laden with major methodological obstacles. When groups of women are surveyed without strict inclusive and exclusive criteria, using only negative questions and retrospective reporting, most of the subjects often qualify for a diagnosis of "premenstrual syndrome." Further contributing to this phenomenon is the considerable currency that the diagnosis has gained in the lay population and media. That symptoms, by definition, are subjective experiences is particularly problematic when society sees certain experiences as normative and when individual psychology and coping are not taken into account (Gallant et al. 1992a, 1992b).

The diagnosis of PMS, or LLPDD, is based on self-reports. Several studies have demonstrated overwhelming discrepancies between women's beliefs that they have PMS and their prospectively reported daily symptoms (McFarlane et al. 1988; Parlee 1982). For example, Ainscough (1990) had 51 subjects complete menstrual distress questionnaires daily for 8 weeks without revealing the purpose of the experiment. Although the prospective data revealed no premenstrual increase in negative affect, most of the subjects retrospectively reported that they had experienced "premenstrual tension" during the course of the study (Ainscough 1990). Many women who report that they have PMS actually have symptoms throughout the menstrual cycle; such women are likely to have had psychiatric treatment and family stress and disruption (West 1989). Prospective daily ratings, then, are more reliable than are retrospective data, but when subjects are not blinded to the purpose of the study, their ratings may be vulnerable to the same bias. People have the symptoms they expect to have and attribute those symptoms to the etiologies their culture accepts (Koeske and Koeske 1975). Women are not blind to their own menstrual status. Some researchers have attempted to correct for this methodologic problem by studying women who have undergone hysterectomies. Such women, however, can still be expected to be made aware of their hormonal cycles by the physical changes of the premenstruum. The vast majority of studies have been performed on women who believe, and often insist, that they have a premenstrual disorder.

The criteria outlined in DSM-III-R were intended to address these problems. In many clinical settings, however, it is difficult to obtain compliance with the required 2 months of prospective daily ratings. When the Work Group on LLPDD sought data from five excellent PMS clinics for reanalysis, only 670 of the 1,089 original subjects had provided sufficient or acceptable information (Hurt et al. 1992). Often the number of subjects who qualify for study is very small. Many studies have not required cessation of symptoms after the onset of menstrual bleeding. No stipulation as to the nature of functional impairment is made. There is some evidence that most or all women experience cyclical variations in mood and that the real difference between those who do and do not report that they have PMS is in their perceptions of and reactions to identical experiences (Gallant et al. 1992a, 1992b).

Most researchers who work with subjects with PMS are not blinded, and appropriate control subjects are not included. No data exist on the clinical use of the diagnosis in the field. Given the amount of time required to plan, obtain funding for, perform, analyze, and publish a scientific study, it is not surprising that as recently as April 1992, a journal article stated that the criteria for LLPDD had been published while the study was in progress (Freeman et al. 1992). At least several more years must elapse before a significant data base using DSM-III-R criteria will have accumulated.

Rigorous definition drastically decreases the number and percentage of defined subjects with LLPDD. Such a difference between those who assert that they have a particular disease or condition in the absence of any objective evidence for it and those who are officially categorized as ill poses a problem for medicine and for society. There is something of an analogous situation in the average ambulatory primary-care setting. Most of the people presenting for care do not have a straightforward medical illness as customarily defined, but have either a diagnosable psychiatric illness or a medical condition complicated and compounded by psychosocial factors (Regier et al. 1978; Schurman et al. 1985). The people without a defined medical disorder tend to be ignored and derided. A rich vocabulary of dismissive and derogatory terms is used to distinguish them from "bona fide" patients. They are "crocks." Will this term be used to characterize the millions of women who do not fulfill rigorous diagnostic criteria for LLPDD?

Studies documented in other chapters of this book have demonstrated that many women who report that they have PMS and who do not fit diagnostic criteria actually have other psychiatric disorders. Unfortunately, clinicians report that some of these women refuse to accept the accurate diagnoses and the appropriate treatment for them. Given a legitimized diagnostic category, a large group of people who wish to receive that diagnosis, and a history of difficulty obtaining adequate data and loose interpretation of criteria, there may be a tremendous temptation for practitioners to use this diagnosis to attract, gratify, and inappropriately treat patients.

Another difficulty is the lack of a specific and effective treatment for premenstrual symptoms. What do we have to offer that small segment of symptomatic women who do qualify for a narrowly defined syndrome? First, there is a good deal of psychic relief in the recognition of symptoms as genuine "disease." Second, almost all studies of treatments demonstrate symptomatic improvement. Perhaps some women are successfully treated for other illnesses mistakenly identified as PMS. Both minor tranquilizers and fluoxetine have been reported to be effective in the treatment of LLPDD. This may argue for premenstrual symptoms as a "calling card" for women who have difficulty coping with stressful lives, and/or for LLPDD as a subset of depressive illness. The treatment literature reveals no replicative and successful hormonal interventions, despite the intrinsic identification of LLPDD as a hormonally related illness.

Several studies report the use of ovariectomy, hysterectomy, and hormonal regimens that completely disrupt the normal menstrual cycle. Although these interventions have been associated with sustained symptomatic improvement in some cases, they are of concern for several reasons. First, female castration has a long historical association with the care of troubled and troubling women. Second, castration has profound psychological meanings and permanent reproductive implications. Male castration invariably occasions much more ethical, social, political, and medical concern and is rarely performed. Third, ablation of organs without demonstrable organic pathology is a rather primitive approach to a psychiatric syndrome. Fourth, the placebo effect of major surgery, especially surgery on the organs the woman believes to be the source of her troubles, can be expected to be considerably larger than the placebo effect of medication or other relatively benign interventions.

Related Nosological Issues

LLPDD, under whatever name, is by definition a hormonally related condition, despite the failure to identify a specific hormonal etiology or treatment to date. Many endocrine aberrations, such as those of the thyroid and adrenal gland, are associated with derangements of mood, cognition, and behavior. It is nosologically lopsided and clumsy to single out one such syndrome as a psychiatric disorder. Furthermore, when the proposed disorder is limited to one gender, it "pathologizes" the physiological functioning of that gender. As indicated above, hormones that are intrinsic to male reproductive function have also been associated with socially destructive behavioral dysfunction but without classification (Dabbs and Morris 1990).

LLPDD is also identified and labeled as a disorder of mood.

There is increasing evidence of its etiologic and therapeutic association with the depressive illnesses. Classification possibilities more intellectually rigorous than a freestanding diagnosis would be a diagnostic code to indicate hormonal concomitants of any psychiatric diagnosis, or a general category of hormonally related disorders.

Conclusions

We return to the questions of the importance of the psychological, social, political, and legal context of psychiatric diagnosis and of the double bind into which the consideration of signs and symptoms related to female reproductive functions puts women. Both of these realities, and our scientific tradition, demand that a proposed psychiatric diagnosis of PMS, by whatever name, be supported by a wealth of well-controlled, prospective data obtained under conditions that scrupulously address and minimize attributional bias on the part of subjects and investigators. They demand that comparable, and more socially devastating, effects of male hormones on the state and behavior of men receive equal diagnostic attention. They demand the conceptual consideration of such a syndrome in parallel without hormonal conditions—as a medical condition, as a part of diagnostic codes for other psychiatric disorders, or separately, as endocrine-related psychiatric entities. We ought not raise the hopes of the millions of women who believe that their symptoms are due to PMS by prematurely implying that a hormonally based disease has been identified and a specific treatment developed. We cannot ignore the possibilities of a medical, psychiatric, social, political, and legal misuse of diagnostic labels, and the effect of that misuse on the status of all women.

References

Ainscough CE: Premenstrual emotional changes: a prospective study of symptomatology in normal women. J Psychosom Res 34:35–45, 1990

American Psychiatric Association: Diagnostic and Statistical Manual of Mental Disorders, 3rd Edition, Revised. Washington, DC, American Psychiatric Association, 1987

Brooks J, Ruble D, Clark A: College women's attitudes and expectations concerning menstrual-related changes. Psychosom Med 98:288–298, 1977

Caplan PJ: How do they decide who is normal? the bizarre, but true, tale of the DSM process. Can J Psychol 32:162–170, 1991

Chait LR: Premenstrual syndrome and our sisters in crime: a feminist dilemma. Women's Rights Law Reporter 9:267–293, 1986

Coughlin PC: Premenstrual syndrome: how marital satisfaction and role choice affect symptom severity. Soc Work 35:351–355, 1990

Dabbs JM Jr, Morris R: Testosterone, social class, and antisocial behavior in a sample of 4,462 men. Psychological Science 1:209–211, 1990

Dalton K: The Menstrual Cycle. New York, Pantheon, 1969

Dalton K: Once a month. Pomona, CA, Hunter House, 1979

Delaney J, Lipton MJ, Toth E: The Curse: A Cultural History of Menstruation. New York, Dutton, 1976

Fabrega H Jr: Cultural relativism and psychiatric illness. J Nerv Ment Dis 177:415–430, 1989

Freeman EW, Rickels K, Sondheimer SJ: Course of premenstrual syndrome symptom severity after treatment. Am J Psychiatry 149:531–533, 1992

Gallant SJ, Popiel DA, Hoffman DM, et al: Using daily ratings to confirm premenstrual syndrome/late luteal phase dysphoric disorder, I: effects of demand characteristics and expectations. Psychosom Med 54(2):149–166, 1992a

Gallant SJ, Popiel DA, Hoffman DM, et al: Using daily ratings to confirm premenstrual syndrome/late luteal phase dysphoric disorder, II: what makes a "real" difference? Psychosom Med 54(2):167–181, 1992b

Hamilton JA, Gallant SA, Lloyd C: Evidence for a menstrual-linked artifact in determining rates of depression. J Nerv Ment Dis 177:359–365, 1989

Harrison W, Endicott J: Characteristics of women seeking treatment for PMS. Psychosomatics 30:405–411, 1989

Hartmann L: Presidential address: reflections on humane values and biopsychosocial integration. Am J Psychiatry 149:1135–1141, 1992

Heilbrun AB Jr, Frank ME: Self-preoccupation and general stress level as sensitizing factors in premenstrual and menstrual distress. J Psychosom Res 33:571–577, 1989

Hellerstein D: The training of a gynecologist: how the "old boys" talk about women's bodies. MS Magazine, November 1984, pp 136–137

Hersey RB: Emotional cycles in man. Journal of Mental Science 77:151–169, 1931

Holtzman E: Premenstrual syndrome as a legal defense, in The Premenstrual Syndromes. Edited by Gise LH, Kase NG, Berkowitz RL. New York, Churchill Livingstone, 1988, pp 137–143

Hurt SW, Schnurr PP, Severino SK, et al: Late luteal phase dysphoric disorder in 670 women evaluated for premenstrual complaints. Am J Psychiatry 149:525–530, 1992

Koeske RK, Koeske GF: An attributional approach to mood and the menstrual cycle. J Pers Soc Psychol 31:473–478, 1975

Kutchins J, Kirk SA: DSM-III-R: the conflict over new psychiatric diagnoses. Health Soc Work 14:91–101, 1989

Laws S: The sexual politics of premenstrual tension. Women's Studies International Forum 6:19–31, 1983

Laws S: Issues of Blood. London, Macmillan, 1990

Lothstein LM: Female sexuality and feminine development: Freud and his legacy. Adv Psychosom Med 12:57–70, 1985

McEwen BS: Basic research perspectives: ovarian hormone influence on brain neurochemical functions, in The Premenstrual Syndromes. Edited by Gise LH, Kase NG, Berkowitz RL. New York, Churchill Livingstone, 1988, pp 21–33

McFarlane J, Martin CL, Williams TM: Mood fluctuations: women versus men and menstrual versus other cycles. Psychology of Women Quarterly 12:201–223, 1988

Metcalf MG, Livesey JH, Wells JE, et al: Mood cyclicity in women with and without the premenstrual syndrome. J Psychosom Res 33:407–418, 1989

Parlee MB: Social and emotional aspects of menstruation, birth and menopause, in Psychosomatic Obstetrics and Gynecology. Edited by Youngs DD, Ehrhardt AA. New York, Appleton-Century-Crofts, 1980, pp 67–79

Parlee MB: Changes in moods and activation levels during the menstrual cycle in experimentally naive subjects. Psychology of Women Quarterly 7:119–131, 1982

Regier DA, Goldberg ID, Taube CA: The de facto US mental health system. Arch Gen Psychiatry 35:685–693, 1978

Reik T: Page Rites in Judaism. New York, Farrar Strauss, 1964

Schurman RA, Kramer PD, Mitchell JB: The hidden mental health network: treatment of mental illness by nonpsychiatrist physicians. Arch Gen Psychiatry 42:89–94, 1985

Scully D, Bart P: A funny thing happened on the way to the orifice: women in gynecology textbooks, in Changing Women in a Changing Society. Edited by Huber J. Chicago, IL, University of Chicago Press, 1973, pp 283–288

Shye D, Jaffe B: Prevalence and correlates of perimenstrual symptoms: a study of Israeli teenage girls. J Adolesc Health 12:217–224, 1991

Stephens WA: A cross-cultural study of menstrual taboos. Genetic Psychology Monographs 64:385–416, 1961

Stewart DE: Positive changes in the premenstrual period. Acta Psychiatr Scand 79:400–405, 1989

Verbrugge LM: Female illness rates and illness behavior. Women Health 4:61–79, 1979

West CP: The characteristics of 100 women presenting to a gynecological clinic with premenstrual complaints. Acta Obstet Gynecol Scand 68:743–747, 1989

Winter EJS, Ashton DJ, Moore DL: Dispelling myths: a study of PMS and relationship satisfaction. Nurse Pract 16:34–45, 1991

Youngs DD, Reame N: Psychoneuroendocrinology and the menstrual cycle, psychosomatic obstetrics and gynecology. Adv Psychosom Med 12:25–34, 1985

❧ 9 ☙

Sociocultural Influences on Women's Experiences of Perimenstrual Symptoms

Alice J. Dan, Ph.D., and
Lisa Monagle, Ph.D., C.N.M.

> [B]iology has never been destiny . . . even those func-
> tions most often described as eternal have always been
> formed by cultural and social organization.
>
> Gordon 1990, p. 475

This book is part of a process of social negotiation about the
nature of the menstrual experience. There are many sides to
this argument and many interest groups, and this chapter cannot hope to examine all of them in sufficient depth. Rather, we
propose to give an interpretation of the process and to provide
examples to illustrate its various facets in order to better understand the impact of social context on women's experience of
symptoms.

Among its other characteristics, the menstrual cycle is a socially
constructed phenomenon (Dan 1986; Johnson 1983; M. B. Parlee,
"The Social Construction of Premenstrual Syndrome: A Case
Study of Discourse as Cultural Contestation," unpublished manuscript, 1992; Rodin 1992). This sociocultural reality exists, with
greater or lesser salience, for all who participate in a society,

whether they menstruate or not. The particular social understanding of menstruation can vary among different societies; at that level, the reality is referred to as *cultural*. The ubiquity of menstruation and its exclusive association with women are major reasons for the social construction of the menstrual experience to occupy a significant place in a society's view of women. Indeed, it has been argued that menstruation is a key marker for women's difference from men and for the interpretation that women are therefore "abnormal" (Fausto-Sterling 1985).

If the menstrual experience is conceptualized as underlying female disability in comparison with males, that concept can be used to legitimate practices that oppress women. Furthermore, it becomes problematic to understand what is normal and what can be disordered in menstrual experience if a society's conceptions of all menstrual phenomena are basically negative. The raging controversies over the existence and nature of perimenstrual symptoms can best be understood not just as scientific debates, but also as a struggle to integrate traditional scientific ways of thinking about the menstrual cycle with insights from recent feminist research.

Because the social context for scientific work influences the focus of research and how questions are asked, it is important to understand how the dominant social reality constructs menstrual phenomena and what alternative constructions might be suggested by women's experiences. For example, the textbook definition of a "normal" menstrual cycle generally includes characteristics related to fertility and particular patterns of hormonal change, even though missed ovulation and a shortened luteal phase are not uncommon variations in women without menstrual cycle complaints. Whether these variations are considered abnormal or symptomatic or as part of the normal range may depend on how salient is the reproductive aspect of menstrual function for an investigator. For most women today, however, reproduction does not constitute the major aspect of menstrual experience. The menstrual cycle as a "normal" phenomenon has been systematically *un*-studied. Women with menstrual cycles have, until very recently, been purposefully omitted from research of all kinds, from heart disease to drug interventions, because the menstrual cycle was viewed as "noise" or "interference."

The process of institutionalizing a particular construction of menstrual experience, as in developing the official DSM diagnoses, requires considerable resources. Because women historically have had less access to resources of all kinds, it is not surprising that current social reality does not adequately reflect the menstrual experience of women.[1] Because we are now more sensitized to the consequences of a lack of symmetry between female experience and institutionalized social reality in general, however, we would propose as a primary goal of this process the creation of a better fit between the proposed social definition and perimenstrual experiences as women live them. The purpose of this chapter is to examine available clues about the influences of social and cultural constructions of premenstrual phenomena that can be gathered from two sources of empirical studies: those indicating social impact within a society and those comparing results across cultures.

Studies of Social Impact

Two kinds of data broadly suggest that the dominant social portrayal of menstrual phenomena is different from how they are experienced. One type of study compares attitudes toward menstruation or menopause of groups with and without the actual experiences. Thus, for example, younger premenarcheal girls have been found to have significantly more negative attitudes toward menstruation than do older, postmenarcheal girls (Brooks-Gunn and Ruble 1980). Similarly, men and premenopausal women have evaluated menopause more negatively than have postmenopausal women (Bowles 1992; Kahana et al. 1980). Parlee (1974) also demonstrated that the beliefs of male college students about the effects of the menstrual cycle on women were

---

[1] Many feminist scholars and theorists have analyzed the discrepancies between socially defined institutions and women's actual or "lived" experience (see, e.g., Haraway 1989; Rich 1976; Schaef 1981).

more negative than were those of their female counterparts.

In the second type of study, comparisons are made between retrospective reports of cyclic symptoms and prospective daily recordings of symptoms. In these studies, the same individuals make these two different kinds of assessments. The findings have consistently shown that a discrepancy exists, with the retrospective reports showing higher symptom levels than the daily recordings (e.g., Shaver and Woods 1985). These two types of evidence, then, appear to indicate the effects of the negative social context for menstrual experiences generally.

On the other hand, because retrospective reflection is still widely used to measure premenstrual symptoms (in fact, it is almost the only measure used in cross-cultural comparisons), it is important to try to understand the reality value of these reports by women of their experiences—not so much in terms of whether they are true or not true, but rather what reality they represent. To what extent is this reality based in normal or pathological physiology of the menstrual cycle? To what extent does it reflect sociocultural beliefs and assumptions? What cognitive or affective mechanisms may result from these findings? To answer these questions, we need to look not only at women who identify themselves as experiencing premenstrual distress (based initially on retrospective reflection), but also at population-based studies to provide a context for understanding. Examples of recent studies illustrating the questions raised by both approaches are presented here.

Taylor and colleagues (1991) reported a study of a population-based sample that included over 600 women. Groups with marked ($n = 222$) and modest ($n = 119$) differences in symptom severity during a particular phase of the menstrual cycle were used to construct and test a causal model predicting the severity of perimenstrual negative affect. The strongest predictors of prospectively measured perimenstrual negative affect were levels of life stress and general distress (as measured on depression and anxiety scales). Socialization to negative expectations of menstruation also significantly contributed to severe perimenopausal negative affect. In addition, these experiences of negative affect showed different patterns than did somatic symptoms, suggesting that negative affect is "a different experience than somatic perimenstrual symptoms" (Taylor et al. 1991, p. 116).

Gallant and colleagues (1992a, 1992b) followed a more common protocol of recruiting volunteers, 35 of whom reported severe premenstrual distress and provisionally met the criteria for late luteal phase dysphoric disorder (LLPDD) and another 35 of whom reported no premenstrual symptoms. When these groups were followed for 2 months with prospective daily ratings of symptoms, they were not as divergent as expected in their symptom reports. Not only were there low symptom reports among those provisionally identified as having premenstrual syndrome (PMS)—which is not an unusual finding (Rubinow et al. 1984)—but also among the women perceiving themselves to have no PMS, some reported premenstrual symptom levels at or higher than the PMS group. In examining what variables would best differentiate the two groups, the investigators found that factors related to low self-esteem, coping patterns, anger, and guilt allowed better discrimination between the groups than did actual cyclic symptom changes. They suggest that cyclic changes should be understood as normative, whereas differences in perception or meanings given to the changes result in distress and identification as an individual with PMS.

Hamilton and Gallant (1993) presented a useful scheme in which the groups to be studied included systematic variation of three factors: 1) retrospective reports of PMS, 2) prospective reports of premenstrual symptoms, and 3) comorbidity. It seems particularly important to include not only those subjects whose retrospective and prospective reports are positive for PMS (with no comorbidity) in comparison with those who report no symptoms retrospectively or prospectively, but also to study the group characterized as experiencing "retrospective PMS" and those who report symptoms prospectively but are not distressed enough by them to consider themselves as having PMS.

Cross-Cultural Studies

In cross-cultural studies, perimenstrual symptom rates have been reported in women of more than 20 different nationalities, with

wide variation in predominant symptoms and levels of symptomatology (Chandra and Chaturvedi 1989; Hasin et al. 1988; Janiger et al. 1972; Snowden and Christian 1983). By far the most
widely used measure is the retrospective Moos Menstrual Distress Questionnaire (MDQ [Moos 1968]); we have seen only one
report of a prospective study (among !Kung women; Hamilton
and Gallant 1993). Recently, a more systematic comparison was
made through similar methodological approaches in three cultures: the United States (Woods et al. 1982), Italy (Monagle
1987), and Bahrain (Al-Gasseer 1990 [Table 9–1]). In all three
of these studies, the authors utilized representative population
samples of community women, who completed the original or
carefully translated versions of the MDQ. Participation rates
among the groups contacted were similar (72%–74% completed
the questionnaires), and the numbers of women participating
ranged from 179 to 239.

The U.S. and Bahraini women were similar in age (27.3 and

Table 9–1. Demographic characteristics of U.S., Bahraini, and Italian subjects

Characteristic	U.S. (Woods et al. 1982) (*n* = 179)	Bahraini (Al-Gasseer 1990) (*n* = 172)	Italian (Monagle 1987) (*n* = 239)
Age (years)			
Mean ± SD	27.3 ± 4.5	28.0 ± 7	35.5 ± 8
Range	18–> 31	17–45	20–45
Race (%)			
White	67	100	100
Black	33	—	—
Education (%)			
High school or less	12	78.0	85.7
Some college	28	20.0	14.3
College graduate or more	60	2.0	0
Religion (%)			
Catholic	11	0	96
Protestant	65	0	0
Jewish, none,			
Jehovah's Witness	24	0	4
Muslim, other	0	100	0

28.0 years, respectively), whereas the Italian women were slightly older on average (35.5 years). The U.S. sample was the only racially diverse sample (33% black, 67% white); the Italian and Bahraini samples exhibited homogeneity with regard to race. The sample of U.S. women was the most highly educated group: 88% of the women reported either some college education or had attained one or more college degrees, whereas only 22% of the Bahraini women and 14.3% of the Italian women reported the same level of educational attainment.

Most of the U.S. women reported their religious affiliation as Protestant, the Bahraini women were exclusively Muslim, and the Italian women were overwhelmingly Catholic. The vast majority of the U.S. women worked outside the home (82%), whereas only 38% of the Bahraini women and 20% of the Italian women did so. The majority of women in all three cultural groups were married, with the U.S. and Bahraini samples having similar rates of married and single women (60% and 32%–40%, respectively). (In the Bahraini married category, however, first, second, and third wives were included, whereas the number of previous marriages among the U.S. women was not listed separately.) The highest proportion of married women was found in the Italian sample, with almost 83% of the women married for the first time at the time of data collection.

With regard to menstrual cycle characteristics, the U.S. and Italian sample's mean age at menarche, cycle lengths, and flow lengths were almost identical. Bahraini women, on the other hand, had a slightly later average age at menarche, with slightly shorter cycle lengths and slightly longer flow lengths than in the U.S. and Italian women.

Few women in Italy or Bahrain reported any knowledge of PMS or premenstrual tension. Most symptoms occurred at significantly different prevalence rates among the three cultures. In general, U.S. and Italian women reported higher symptom prevalence rates than did Bahraini women. Five symptoms emerged as consistently reported in 30% or more of the women during the premenstrual phase, in all three cultures: swelling, 38%–64%; irritability, 32%–56%; breast pain, 35%–54%; mood swings, 36%–51%; and fatigue,

32%–34%. Irritability and mood swings were significantly more prevalent among U.S. women than among Italian or Bahraini women. Among the top five most frequently experienced symptoms for U.S. women were tension and weight gain. Among the Italian women, swelling and breast pain were experienced by significantly more women than in the other two groups, whereas other frequently experienced symptoms (among the top five) were tension and backache. The most frequent symptom among Bahrainian women was backache (experienced by 49%).

Symptom clusters found consistently across all three cultures, through factor analysis, were those of negative affect (including tension, anxiety, irritability, mood swings), water retention (swelling, painful breasts), and decreased activity (taking naps, fatigue). A symptom cluster found to be exclusively reported by Italian women was premenstrual well-being (full of energy and well-being, orderliness).

These studies across three cultures support the interpretation that cyclic change is normative, while also showing how systematic differences characterize each culture. Studies in the United States suggest the importance of comorbidity of patterns of interpretation and/or behavior that apparently increase vulnerability to the negative impact of premenstrual changes. In general, the same kind of information is not available from other cultures. This is, therefore, an important area of investigation that would greatly increase our understanding of premenstrual symptom experience. It will be especially useful to compare situations in which definitions of PMS (or premenstrual dysphoric disorder) become available and most women are aware of them with situations in which these are not cultural categories. Prospective as well as retrospective data are needed from a variety of cultures.

Conclusions

Developing a social reality takes time, sharing of experiences, and access to resources. The PMS action groups of the 1970s and 1980s are an example of this process, but it is not clear what role their activities have played in the total picture. A great deal of caution is advocated in this process of institutionalizing definitions of menstrual experience, because whatever definitions are developed will operate within the larger system, which is still dominated by male perspectives. The potential, therefore, of "pathologizing" a normal female experience or perpetuating negative stereotypes is dangerous. Furthermore, despite the best intentions of those seeking to formally legitimate women's premenstrual experiences, the consequences are unpredictable, as has been found with affirmative action and no-fault divorce. Sometimes what looks like a useful solution or compromise turns out to work against us. Perhaps the most important characteristic of a useful conceptualization is its flexibility, so that it can encompass the varieties of experience we are likely to discover.

References

Al-Gasseer J: Perimenopausal symptoms among Bahraini women. Doctoral dissertation, University of Illinois at Chicago, 1990

Bowles C: The development of a measure of attitude toward menopause, in Menstrual Health in Women's Lives. Edited by Dan AJ, Lewis LL. Chicago, University of Illinois Press, 1992, pp 206–212

Brooks-Gunn J, Ruble D: Menarche: the interaction of physiological, cultural, and social factors, in The Menstrual Cyle: A Synthesis of Interdisciplinary Research. Edited by Dan AJ, Graham EA, Beecher CP. New York, Springer, 1980, pp 141–159

Chandra PS, Chaturvedi SK: Cultural variations of premenstrual experience. Int J Soc Psychiatry 35:343–349, 1989

Dan AJ: The law and women's bodies: the case of menstruation leave in Japan. Health Care for Women International 7:1–14, 1986

Fausto-Sterling A: Myths of Gender: Biological Theories About Women and Men. New York, Basic Books, 1985

Gallant SJ, Popiel DA, Hoffman DM, et al: Using daily ratings to confirm premenstrual syndrome/late luteal phase dysphoric disorder, I: effects of demand characteristics and expectations. Psychosom Med 54(2):149–166, 1992a

Gallant SJ, Popiel DA, Hoffman DM, et al: Using daily ratings to confirm premenstrual syndrome/late luteal phase dysphoric disorder, II: what makes a "real" difference? Psychosom Med 54(2):167–181, 1992b

Gordon L: Woman's Body, Woman's Right. New York, Penguin Books, 1990

Hamilton J, Gallant S: Premenstrual syndromes: a health psychology critique of biomedically oriented research, in Psychophysiological Disorders: Research and Clinical Applications. Edited by Gatchel RJ, Blanchard EB. Washington, DC, American Psychological Association, 1993

Haraway D: Primate Visions: Gender, Race and Nature in the World of Modern Science. New York, Routledge, 1989

Hasin M, Dennerstein L, Gotts G: Menstrual cycle related complaints: a cross cultural study. Journal of Psychosomatic Obstetrics and Gynecology 9:35–42, 1988

Janiger O, Riffenburgh R, Kersh K: Cross-cultural study of premenstrual syndrome. Psychosomatics 13:226–235, 1972

Johnson TM: Premenstrual syndrome as a western culture-specific disorder. Cult Med Psychiatry 11:337–356, 1983

Kahana E, Kiyak A, Liang J: Menopause in the context of other life events, in The Menstrual Cycle: A Synthesis of Interdisciplinary Research. Edited by Dan AJ, Graham EA, Beecher CP. New York, Springer, 1980, 167–178

Monagle L: Perimenopausal symptom prevalence among southern Italian women. Doctoral dissertation, University of Illinois at Chicago, 1987

Moos RH: The development of a menstrual distress questionnaire. Psychosom Med 30:853–867, 1968

Parlee MB: Stereotypic beliefs about menstruation—a methodological note on the Moos Menstrual Distress Questionnaire and some new data. Psychosom Med 36:229–440, 1974

Rich A: Of Women Born. New York, Norton, 1976

Rodin M: The social construction of premenstrual syndrome. Soc Sci Med 35:49–56, 1992

Rubinow D, Roy-Byrne P, Hoban MC, et al: Prospective assessment of menstrually related mood disorders. Am J Psychiatry 141:684–686, 1984

Schaef AW: Women's Reality. Minneapolis, MN, Winston Press, 1981

Shaver JF, Woods NF: Concordance of perimenstrual symptoms across two cycles. Res Nurs Health 8:313–319, 1985

Snowden R, Christian B (eds): Patterns and Perceptions of Menstruation: A World Health Organization International Collaborative Study. New York, St. Martins Press, 1983

Taylor D, Woods NF, Lentz MJ, et al: Perimenstrual negative affect: development and testing of an explanatory model, in Menstruation, Health, and Illness. Edited by Taylor DT, Woods NF. New York, Hemisphere, 1991, pp 103–118

Woods NF, Most A, Dery GK: Prevalence of perimenstrual symptoms. Am J Public Health 72:1257–1264, 1982

☙ 10 ❧

Commentary: Late Luteal Phase Dysphoric Disorder—Disease or Dis-Ease?

Sally K. Severino, M.D.

[I]n a complex field, with many simultaneously active variables, and different levels of research and clinical access, continual back and forth motion between analysis and synthesis seems to me essential. So does some *extra* effort to study what is *hard* to study and *long* to study, not just what is relatively easy and fast to quantify and publish. Cooperation and tolerance of complexity seem to me hard but essential in a complex field like brain plus mind plus influences on brain and mind that result in health and illness.

Hartmann 1992, p. 1139

This is a chapter about myths. Myths reflect our beliefs about how and why we were created as man and as woman. To the extent that they transform the unknown in our experience into the known of our nature, they bring certainty to uncertainty and understanding to confusion. In so doing, they provide a means of managing feelings that results in a sense of security. Myths develop out of historical necessity. They then become institutionalized so that they pervade all aspects of life, including family, religion, art, and politics, where they provide us with the security that comes from the sense that we are living in agreement with our beliefs. Myths continue unchanged as long as they provide a sense of security to the majority of the individuals in a culture.

Western civilization has evolved as a patriarchal society (Lerner 1986). The patriarchal conceptual model for the relationship of women to men is one of subordination, and the patriarchal structural model expressing this concept is the tripartite family with man as head and woman and child as subordinates (Lerner 1986). Myths expressing the concept of woman as subordinate to man are so much a part of Western language, institutions, and values that both men and women have difficulty recognizing the inequality, questioning it, understanding it, or changing it (Lerner 1986; MacKinnon 1982). Social changes, however, are forcing a new understanding. Family structure is changing, as evidenced by the fact that fewer than 10% of U.S. families fit the "traditional" model (Nadelson and Notman 1991). Most are characterized by other models, including patterns such as single parents of either sex, non-related adults with and without children, gay couples with and without children, and married couples with children from previous marriages. Women are moving out of the home into the workplace. About two-thirds of all mothers, more than 70% of women with school-age children, and 56% of women with preschool children work outside the home (Jackson 1992; Women's Political Action Group 1992). In addition to these social changes, scientists are contributing to a new appreciation of women's development that will be described later in this chapter and to new understandings of women's biology (see Chapters 3–5).

These forces are demanding a revision of the patriarchal myths, a revision of the conceptual model from a male-led society to a male-female–led society, and a revision of the tripartite family structure to man-woman head with child as dependent. The elementary unit for the conceptual model of society requires three basic elements: a man (sperm), a woman (egg), and the child. They exist in relationships that are elaborations of the basic unit. The myths elaborated from a view of the basic unit of three that sees man as dominant will differ from the myths elaborated from a view of man and woman as dominant. The former view generates the myths perpetuating a patriarchal society, whereas the latter view is necessary to create the myths that will sustain a partnership society.

In this chapter, I describe a simplified version of how the myth of women's subordination to men derives from historical necessity and how this myth is elaborated in our institutions perpetuating history. I describe some of the evolving understanding of women's development across the life cycle that generates questions about the existing myths associated with women and conclude with the questions that this raises about our understanding of the diagnosis of late luteal phase dysphoric disorder (LLPDD).

Origin and Elaboration of Myth

Our myths were based and elaborated upon historically determined gender roles (Rosaldo and Lamphere 1974). A role is the set of behavioral expectations for a person who performs a particular social function (Shaver 1977). Women biologically bore children and of necessity assumed the role of caregiver. Men biologically were stronger and assumed the role of providers. These gender roles became elaborated in myths such as the belief that motherhood is woman's chief goal in life (Warner 1983) and that strength is a sign of man's natural superiority (Lerner 1986). The early laws (cf. coverture [Baker 1979, p. 395] and paterfamilias [Wolff 1951]) that were established to protect the provider's property rights reflected this social structure to the extent that a wife and children were considered the property of the provider, that is, of the man (Eisler 1987).

The principle of man's class status as determined by his economic relations and woman's class status as determined by her sexual relations became elaborated in many different instances (Lerner 1986). For example, in lower-class families, marriage by purchase was economically advantageous, a virgin daughter bringing the highest price. In upper-class families, marriages were used to gain social and economic power. Fathers could also gain spiritual and economic advantage by dedicating daughters to the service of the temple. The Judeo-Christian religion perpetuated the belief that woman is subordinate to man because God created her so (Eisler 1987; Lerner 1986; Ostling 1991; Ranke-Heinemann 1990; Warner 1983).

In other words, historically, men and women accepted a division of labor where women became mothers and child-rearers because it was perceived as functional and survival depended on it (Lerner 1986). These roles and behaviors moved from private practice to public laws and customs that enforced a subordination of women to men. The subordination of women to men became elaborated in myth and religious beliefs that reified women's self-giving tendencies in cultural stereotypes (Ulanov 1975) and attitudes that are powerfully resistant to change, not only on a societal and institutional level, but also within individual men and women.

Many women and men are no longer satisfied with these historical roles. Attempts to assume different roles, however, generate conflicts with the attitudes, feelings, expectations, and meanings that constitute the essence of the self. The self evolves in the context of social relations that regulate and are regulated by the infant's affect and behavior (Sroufe 1989). Ultimately, social relations are a product of the interaction of individuals with the cultural norms that are reflected in their cultural myths. Let us turn, then, to the questions about our cultural myths that arise as our understanding of women's development evolves.

Myth and Women's Development

The literature is replete with data about the influence of nature versus the influence of nurture on women's development, all of which must be rethought (Nadelson et al. 1991; Rosaldo and Lamphere 1974):

> From the moment of conception, nature (biology) and nurture (environment) *interact* with each other so that their relative contributions become virtually inseparable. (Heide 1985, p. 25)

Hormones exert organizational effects on mood and sexuality that can occur prenatally and permanently, as well as activational effects that can be immediate and reversible:

> [E]xperiences—either minute experiences or developmental experiences like sensory input—affect the structure of the brain. Similarly, the structure of the brain and the patterns of transmission and so forth have a profound effect on behavior and on emotional response. . . . (Nadelson et al. 1991, p. 2)

Women's development, then, must be conceptualized in the context of the interaction of nature and nurture. This is a more complex interactive conceptual model.

Infants need caretakers for survival. Girls will identify with the first important caretaker in their lives. If this is a woman, they will learn her way of being female in that particular culture. Their identity will develop as a sense of being continuous with others, a sense of connectedness (Lerner 1986). This continuing sense of connection promotes a process of differentiation to interdependence in an expanding network of connections. These girls will need to learn that separation can be protective as well as isolating (Benjamin 1988; Gilligan 1982). If changing family constellations are such that the girls' first important caretaker is a man, these girls will have to move away from the man to find an identification with a woman in order to learn the way in which women exist in their culture. Their identity will develop as a sense of "other-than-the-man," a sense of separateness (Lerner 1986). This primary separation, linked to disappointment and anger about having to separate, promotes a process of aggressive feelings leading to separation. These girls will need to learn that others are equal and connections are safe (Gilligan 1982). In both situations, it is the process of development that is important (Nadelson et al. 1991).

The first important caretaker will be experienced by the helpless infant as all-powerful and will become associated with fears of powerlessness. He or she will also be the source of peak affect states that the girl will experience as extremely desirable and want to repeat or as extremely undesirable and wish to avoid (Kernberg 1990, p. 125). These affect states organize experience:

> Affects thus can be seen as complex psychic structures that are indissolubly linked to the individual's cognitive appraisals of his immediate situation, and that contain a positive or negative valence with regard to the relation of the subject to the object of the particular experience. (Kernberg 1990, p. 125)

Affects are the consequences of and contributors to ideas (Horowitz 1987):

> Affective organization is repeatedly transformed through biobehavioral shifts . . . as autonomy and individuation increase. (Sameroff and Emde 1989, p. 11)

Contemporary research in infants seems to indicate that positive emotional experiences are organized by the left anterior hemisphere, separately from negative emotional experiences, which are organized by the right anterior hemisphere (Emde 1991).

These specific lived moments constitute the building blocks from which the self develops. The self is "an inner organization of attitudes, feelings, expectations, and meanings that arises from an organized caregiving matrix" (Sroufe 1989, p. 96). Daniel Stern (1989) provides a conceptual model for how these lived moments become represented in the individual's mind, where they determine the individual's behavior. First, the specific lived moments become memories and generalized representations of the moments. Representations of these scenarios then become internal preverbal working models that can become narrative models once the child learns to speak. This conceptual model is important, because it provides a way of explaining how our past relationships become part of the self and determine how we behave in relation to others.

The family is the institution in which the task of growth and development of each member occurs. The behavior of each member is defined by the roles he or she is assigned (Shapiro and Carr

1991). Different kinds of roles exist. Kinship roles define who is mother, father, daughter, son, sister, or brother. Gender identification roles define who is a girl and who is a boy. Gender identity is thought to be well established by age 18 months (Nadelson et al. 1991). Stereotyped roles define who is nurturer, housekeeper, breadwinner, disciplinarian, and so on, and reflect society's shared beliefs that are taught to each generation, constantly reinforcing the system. Irrational roles define the good mother, bad mother, good father, bad father, rebellious teenager, and others, and are created by unconscious conflicts and shared fantasies among the family members (Shapiro and Carr 1991). The family is the setting in which the girl will learn her roles, observe relationships, and begin to construct her beliefs about women's roles and relationships to men (Bayes and Newton 1978). To the extent that she learns to equate masculinity with dominance and femininity with subordination, she will perpetuate patriarchal myths in her relationships with men (Eisler 1987).

The individual woman, then, must be understood in the context of the interaction of her genetic inheritance and her environmental inheritance:

> Internally, biological development is regulated by the genotype to provide a basis for behavioral organization. Externally, an environtype carries the developmental agenda of society, the family, and the parental figure . . . [relationships] become the primary source of variation in early socio-emotional development. (Sameroff and Emde 1989, p. 11)

There are two basic biological differences between women and men: 1) anatomical differences that give rise to self-concepts and 2) physiological differences that give rise to sense of timing:

> If sexual physiology provides the pattern for our experience of the world, what is woman's basic metaphor? It is mystery, *the hidden* . . . [resulting in a] toleration for ambiguity, which they learn from their inability to learn about their own bodies. Women accept limited knowledge as their natural condition. . . . (Paglia 1990, p. 22)

The girl's anatomy gives rise to a self-concept of sensitivity to be-ginnings and endings as experienced in monthly menstrual cy-cles, menarche-menopause, and pregnancy-parturition. Her anatomy generates a sense of finiteness, that is, she has a limited amount of time to bear children. Her reproductive cycle orga-nizes her life. The self-concept of sensitivity lends itself to the development of potential strengths and weaknesses. To the ex-tent that it fosters acceptance, it can lead to the ability to define limits and boundaries. On the other hand, to the extent that it fosters a sense of vulnerability, it can become the foundation upon which the myth of women as subordinate to men is elabo-rated and maintained. Although I will not focus on how men view and respond to these aspects of womanhood, I acknowledge that men and women negotiate a dynamic fit, a complementar-ity. Hence, new understandings of women will demand changes in male-female relationships. If the myth of women as subordi-nate to men changes, it may require men to redefine their self-concepts in terms of their own sense of vulnerability.

By the end of the second year of life, children show a sensitivity to another's distress. In the third year, a sense of togetherness ap-pears, setting the stage for moral development of equity and fair-ness. By age 4, children have learned to share. This process of early moral development is mediated by positive emotions that appear, develop, and expand through interactions between children and caregivers from very early in life. The reciprocal shared looking, smiling, and cooing between infant and caregiver grows into the moral choice of sharing because of the sought-after affect of joy in bringing pleasure to the other person:

> [T]he extent to which later individual differences in positive emotions represent continuities with early individual differences and positive emotions—either from temperament or from early caregiving experiences—remains an open question. (Emde 1991, p. 24)

The later differences, for example, may reflect the impact of cul-tural beliefs on the individual's temperament or early caretaking experiences. To the extent that early caregiving experiences foster the cultural ideal of caring as womanly and good, this ideal carries the potential for promoting stereotypes of "caring as womanly" and a "good woman as selfless and self-sacrificing." Both of these stereotypes fit dynamically into the myth of women's subordinate position. It is likely that the myth of women's subordinate position and sex role stereotypes of women's self-giving nature need constant reinforcement to perpetuate them and will need early and constant reeducation to change them:

> [W]hile society may affirm publicly the woman's right to choose for herself, the exercise of such choice brings her privately into conflict with the conventions of femininity, particularly the moral equation of goodness with self-sacrifice. (Gilligan 1982, p. 70)

Self-giving is often not assessed in terms of the intentions of the woman and the consequences of the behavior, but on the basis of its appearance in the eyes of others as true femininity (Gilligan 1982). Self-giving is often projected onto particular settings and reified in cultural stereotypes:

> The self-giving tendency in a woman [is] projected onto and identified with her having a family, being a wife or a mother, giving herself to others almost entirely in a home setting. [Likewise], [t]he self-fulfilling tendency [is] by and large projected onto and reified in the image of woman fulfilling herself through a career, a job, a self-conscious moving out into the world. (Ulanov 1975, p. 12)

When women request assessment for their behavior, it threatens men and women who believe in the cultural stereotypes, and it threatens institutions that promote as truth the myth that femininity is self-giving. It is in this context that the images of women derived from the Virgin Mary (Ostling 1991; Warner 1983) and gender differences in the description of God (Schoenfeld and Mestrovic 1991) are being questioned.

From ages 5 through 15, girls socialize by playing in small groups or pairs cooperatively, using talk to cement the relationships (Tannen 1986). Puberty is a time of elaboration of gender identity and a vulnerable time for girls (Nadelson et al. 1991). Girls become less certain and unsure of what they can say without being called stupid or rude. They struggle with self-esteem:

> [P]ersonal doubts . . . invade women's sense of themselves, compromising their ability to act on their own perceptions and thus their willingness to take responsibility for what they do. (Gilligan 1982, p. 49)

A woman's identity is completed with intimacy.

The ideas of predictable progress through adulthood, concepts of psychological normality, and beliefs about normal patterns of behavior for women are changing. The concept of stages of development seems unsuitable for women because the interaction of age with life task varies tremendously among women (Nadelson et al. 1991). We lack norms for women. It is no longer "truth" that middle age for women is, of necessity, accompanied by depression. We lack measures of health for women. The former notion of health consisting of a good adjustment to one's environment makes women victims of the myth of subordination and the sex role stereotypes that are derivative of it (Broverman et al. 1970).

An individual woman, then, develops multiple self-concepts (Horowitz 1987). Flax (1987) has described three self-concepts of women: 1) the social self, 2) the sexual self, and 3) the autonomous self, which she clearly delineates in terms of what is expressed and what is repressed in reaction to societal pressures. What is becoming increasingly appreciated is how multidetermined are the changes required of an individual woman continuously throughout life:

> Every period of life brings new demands; maturational unfolding does not end with adolescence, and cultural shifts undermine or reinforce certain roles. It is never possible to say for sure that a given alteration in behavior was due to a particular change force; every outcome [is] pluridetermined. (Horowitz 1987, p. 150)

Given this evolving understanding of women's development in the context of the patriarchal myth of women's subordination to men, let us begin to explore the contemporary interest in the condition popularly known as premenstrual syndrome (PMS).

Myths and PMS/LLPDD

Certain myths about women interface with the belief that menstruation is related to illness. These myths include 1) all women are fundamentally more emotionally labile than men, especially around the time of their menses, and 2) all women are more difficult to live with premenstrually.

In the context of such ancient myths, various labels have been given to women who complain of premenstrual symptoms: PMS, premenstrual tension, premenstrual tension syndrome, LLPDD, and premenstrual dysphoric disorder (PMDD). Why such difficulty deciding on a name for a condition? To find the answer, we must look at our values. Values result from our biology and our culture and determine what we see and how we see it. Values form the basis of our convictions. We are in an age that demands that we change our convictions about women. Change is threatening.

The difficulty in deciding on a name reflects the difficulty we are having in understanding women and in changing our values. On one level, to those who value "nosology," the threat is losing a psychiatric diagnosis they believe in, so they fight for classification. To those who value "women's rights," the threat is losing credibility, so they fight against stigmatization. Both are right, and both are wrong to the extent that their view is only a portion of the total picture. Both want to help women. The fight should be not to crush each other's views, but to support each other as we develop new convictions. We must negotiate a name and a process for understanding the condition that is acceptable to all those threatened by the change, while not sacrificing the goal of understanding and helping women.

This is not an easy task. It is not an easy task because "nosology" and "women's rights" are only the surface manifestations of profound convictions about psychiatry and women that are being questioned. Selecting a name is one small but important part of understanding the biological and cultural conditions that both create our convictions and hold them in place. That so much time and attention is given to this name and this condition is a reflection of its importance as part of a process to develop a new "reality" for women (and men).

It is in the context of these profound convictions that the diagnoses of PMS and LLPDD have, in the past decade, become acceptable topics for discussion in public (Laws 1990). Contributing to this acceptance, women have become more confident as a result of their experiences in managing the addition of career responsibilities to their responsibilities of home and children. This confidence allows them to express their wishes to be understood and allows them to tolerate the criticism of their requests by those who are angered by their demands and frightened about their growing autonomy. On the other hand, rapid social changes have produced changes in women's roles that have resulted in new conflicts, both for women as they accept the new roles and for men as they adjust to women assuming new roles.

These conflicts force a new examination of gender issues. What better focus for beginning such an examination than the menstrual cycle, the biological basis for gender issues! The diagnoses of PMS and LLPDD, then, serve as society's excuse for women to ask for help and understanding. Additionally, they serve as avenues for men to channel their complaints about women and to voice their attitudes about the changes. This fosters a confrontation with and understanding of old attitudes, stereotypes, and myths about women.

For this to occur, however, PMS and LLPDD must be named and defined. That has been the focus of the DSM process, both for DSM-III-R (American Psychiatric Association 1987) and DSM-IV. Select a name. Describe the condition in terms of symptoms, signs in manifest behavior, and conscious experience of it, both by the woman and the significant others in her life. Then the condition can be studied.

It must be studied from many perspectives. The biological perspective has been the major focus of physicians. PMS and LLPDD, however, must be studied from other perspectives. Johnson (1987) has hypothesized that PMS is a culture-specific syndrome. As such, it expresses key elements of society's structures, such as its statuses, relationships, and institutions, as well as the cultural beliefs upon which these elements exist:

> Viewed as a culture-specific syndrome, PMS is an appropriate symbolic representation of conflicting societal expectations that women be both productive and reproductive. By simultaneously denying either alternative, PMS translates role conflict into a standardized cultural idiom. (Johnson 1987, p. 337)

In other words, the cultural idiom accepts PMS as a legitimate condition (i.e., the woman has PMS) as well as one that denies that the woman is productive (i.e., she is too sick to work) and that she is reproductive (i.e., she is not pregnant):

> Not only can culture-bound syndromes "represent alternative structural possibilities in ritual form, [they] can develop into counterstructure that can actively introduce changes in existing social structure" . . . . In short, a culture-bound syndrome can serve as a symbolic mechanism for both structural maintenance and change in a particular society and, so studied, can assist in the identification and understanding of salient cultural upheavals. (Johnson 1987, p. 348)

> PMS serves to answer this role conflict of productivity and generativity by simultaneously and symbolically denying the possibility of each: in menstruating, one is potentially fertile but obviously non-pregnant; in having incapacitating symptomatology one is exempted from normal work role expectations. With PMS, women can be seen as "victims" who did not "choose" to be sick. Through PMS, Western culture translates the ambiguous and conflicted status of women into a standardized cultural idiom which makes her position "meaningful." It is a symbolic cultural "safety valve" which recognizes the need for women to simultaneously turn away from *either* alternative role demand. (Johnson 1987, p. 349)

By defining women as potentially "in control" of heretofore de-
valued constitutional characteristics, PMS "negotiates" access to
power in a way which indirectly legitimatizes the changing status
of women without directly threatening or destroying the structural status quo. (Johnson 1987, p. 350)

We must, then, study the interaction of culture and attitudes
about menstruation (Chandra and Chaturvedi 1992; Furth and
Shu-Yueh 1992).

At least 24 countries have published studies of PMS (Tucker
and Whalen 1991). These represent opportunities to study PMS
and LLPDD as reflections of particular cultural stereotypes (Hardie and McMurray 1992; McFarland et al. 1989), as expressions of
myths about the menstrual cycle (Achterberg 1991; Bennis and
Nanus 1985; Berry 1988; Caplan et al. 1992; Eagly et al. 1992; Guttman 1983; Rose 1983; Rosenwald and Weirsma 1983; Walker 1992;
White 1967), and as barometers of status and role changes in modern society (Johnson 1987; McSwain 1992; Watson 1992). This includes studying PMS and LLPDD from sociopolitical perspectives
as well (Bernard 1981; Flax 1987; Futterman et al. 1992; Lerner
1986; Miller 1986; Ulanov 1986) and from religious perspectives
(Warner 1983).

Last, but by no means least, PMS and LLPDD must be studied
from the personal perspective to delineate how they reflect an individual woman's development in terms of her physical experience
of menstrual cycle events, her cognitive interpretation of these sen-
sations, her conscious and unconscious emotional responses to
them, and her adaptive behaviors toward them (Wright et al.
1992). What basic needs is a woman fulfilling through her adaptive
behaviors (Rosenwald and Wiersma 1983)? How do these interact
with the personal perspectives of the significant men in the
woman's life, since "[b]oth men's and women's sense of gender and
self partially grow out of and are dependent upon the repression of
women's desire and ambition" (Flax 1987, p. 92)? Both men and
women and their social institutions need study in relation to the
personal experience, because all will be affected and changed by
the understanding derived from the study (Shapiro and Carr 1991).

This is the context surrounding the review of literature conducted by the members of the American Psychiatric Association DSM-IV Work Group on LLPDD, and this is the spirit in which I encourage the continuation of the process of labeling, describing, studying, and learning.

References

Achterberg J: Woman as Healer. Boston, MA, Shambhala, 1991

American Psychiatric Association: Diagnostic and Statistical Manual of Mental Disorders, 3rd Edition, Revised. Washington, DC, American Psychiatric Association, 1987

Baker JH: An Introduction to English Legal History. London, Butterworth, 1979

Bayes M, Newton PM: Women in authority: a sociopsychological analysis. Journal of Applied Behavioral Science 14:7–20, 1978

Benjamin J: The Bonds of Love: Psychoanalysis, Feminism and the Problems of Domination. New York, Pantheon, 1988

Bennis W, Nanus B: Leaders: The Strategies for Taking Charge. New York, Harper & Row, 1985

Bernard J: The Female World. New York, Free Press, 1981

Berry T: The Dream of the Earth. San Francisco, CA, Sierra Club Books, 1988

Broverman IK, Broverman DM, Clarkson FE, et al: Sex-role stereotypes and clinical judgements of mental health. J Consult Clin Psychol 34:1–7, 1970

Caplan PJ, McCurdy-Myers J, Gans M: Should "premenstrual syndrome" be called a psychiatric abnormality? Feminism and Psychology 2:27–44, 1992

Chandra PS, Chaturvedi SK: Cultural variations in attitudes toward menstruation. Can J Psychiatry 37:196–198, 1992

Eagly AH, Makhijami MG, Klonsky BC: Gender and the evaluation of leaders: a meta-analysis. Psychol Bull 111:3–22, 1992

Eisler R: The Chalice and the Blade. New York, HarperCollins, 1987

Emde RN: Positive emotions for psychoanalytic theory: surprises from infancy research and new directions. J Am Psychoanal Assoc 39:5–44, 1991

Flax J: Re-membering the selves: is the repressed gendered? Michigan Quarterly Review 26:92–110, 1987

Furth C, Shu-Yueh C: Chinese medicine and the anthropology of menstruation in contemporary Taiwan. Medical Anthropology 6:27–48, 1992

Futterman LA, Jones JE, Miccio-Fonseca LC, et al: Severity of premenstrual symptoms in relation to medical/psychiatric problems and life experiences. Percept Mot Skills 74:787–799, 1992

Gilligan C: In a Different Voice: Psychological Theory and Women's Development. Cambridge, MA, Harvard University Press, 1982

Guttman HA: Autonomy and motherhood. Psychiatry 48:230–234, 1983

Hardie EA, McMurray NE: Self-stereotyping, sex role ideology, and menstrual attitudes: a social identity approach. Sex Roles 27:17–37, 1992

Hartmann L: Presidential address: reflections on humane values and biopsychosocial integration. Am J Psychiatry 149:1135–1141, 1992

Heide WS: Feminism for the Health of It. New York, Margaretdaughters, 1985

Horowitz MJ: States of Mind. New York, Plenum, 1987

Jackson D: How to Make the World a Better Place for Women. New York, Hyperion, 1992

Johnson TM: Premenstrual syndrome as a Western culture–specific disorder. Cult Med Psychiatry 11:337–356, 1987

Kernberg O: New perspectives in psychoanalytic affect theory, in Emotion: Theory, Research and Experience, Vol 5. Edited by Plutchik R, Kellerman H. New York, Academic Press, 1990, pp 115–131

Laws S: Issues of Blood: The Politics of Menstruation. London, Macmillan, 1990

Lerner G: The Creation of Patriarchy. New York, Oxford University Press, 1986

MacKinnon CA: Feminism, Marxism, method, and the state: an agenda for theory. Signs: Journal of Women in Culture and Society 7:515–544, 1982

McFarland C, Ross M, DeCourville N: Women's theories of menstruation and biases in recall of menstrual symptoms. J Pers Soc Psychol 57:522–531, 1989

McSwain BS: A conversation with Nancy J. Chodorow. American Psychoanalyst 26:16–26, 1992

Miller JB: Toward a New Psychology of Women. Boston, MA, Beacon Press, 1986

Nadelson CC, Notman MT: The impact of the new psychology of men and women on psychotherapy, in American Psychiatric Press Review of Psychiatry, Vol 10. Edited by Tasman A, Goldfinger SM. Washington, DC, American Psychiatric Press, 1991, pp 608–626

Nadelson CC, Dickstein LJ, Notman MT: Gender issues in psychotherapy, in American College of Psychiatrists (ACP) Psychiatry Update, Vol 11, No 7. Edited by Usdin G. Port Washington, NY, Medical Information Systems, 1991, pp 1–10

Ostling RN: Handmaid or feminist? Time, December 30, 1991, pp 62–66

Paglia C: Sexual Personae. New Haven, CT, Yale University Press, 1990

Ranke-Heinemann V: Eunuchs for the Kingdom of Heaven: Women, Sexuality and the Catholic Church. New York, Doubleday, 1990

Rosaldo M, Lamphere L (eds): Women, Culture and Society. Stanford, CA, Stanford University Press, 1974

Rose H: Hand, brain, and heart: a feminist epistemology for the natural sciences. Signs: Journal of Women in Culture and Society 9:73–90, 1983

Rosenwald GC, Wiersma J: Women, career changes, and the new self: an analysis of rhetoric. Psychiatry 46:213–229, 1983

Sameroff AJ, Emde RN (eds): Relationship Disturbances in Early Childhood: A Developmental Approach. New York, Basic Books, 1989

Schoenfeld E, Mestrovic SG: With justice and mercy: instrumental-masculine and expressive-feminine elements in religion. Journal for the Scientific Study of Religion 30:363–380, 1991

Shapiro ER, Carr AW: Lost in Familiar Places. New Haven, CT, Yale University Press, 1991

Shaver KC: Principles of Social Psychology. Cambridge, MA, Winthrop, 1977

Sroufe LA: Relationships, self, and individual adaptation, in Relationship Disturbances in Early Childhood: A Developmental Approach. Edited by Sameroff AJ, Emde RN. New York, Basic Books, 1989, pp 70–96

Stern DN: The representation of rational patterns: developmental considerations, in Relationship Disturbances in Early Childhood: A Developmental Approach. Edited by Sameroff AJ, Emde RN. New York, Basic Books, 1989, pp 52–69

Tannen D: That's Not What I Meant. New York, Random House, 1986

Tucker JS, Whalen RE: Premenstrual syndrome. Int J Psychiatry Med 21:311–341, 1991

Ulanov AB: The feminine and the world of CPE. Journal of Pastoral Care 29:11–22, 1975

Ulanov AB: For better and for worse. Psychoanal Rev 73:618–620, 1986

Walker A: Men's and women's beliefs about the influence of the menstrual cycle on academic performance: a preliminary study. Journal of Applied Social Psychology 22:896–909, 1992

Warner M: Alone of All Her Sex. New York, Vintage Books, 1983

Watson B: Salem's dark hour: did the devil make them do it? Smithsonian 23:117–131, 1992

White L Jr: The historical roots of our ecologic crisis. Science 155:1203–1207, 1967

Wolff HJ: Roman Law: An Historical Introduction. Norman, OK, University of Oklahoma Press, 1951

Women's Political Action Group: The Women's 1992 Voting Guide: How to Make Your Vote Count. Berkeley, CA, Earth Works Press, 1992

Wright JH, Clark DM, Thase ME: Cognitive therapy of depression and anxiety, in American College of Psychiatrists (ACP) Update, Vol 12. Edited by Usdin G. Port Washington, NY, Medical Information Systems, 1992, pp 1–10

✌ 11 ✌

Summation

Sally K. Severino, M.D., and Judith H. Gold, M.D., F.R.C.P.C.

> At the level of sensation, your images and my images are virtually the same. . . . Beyond that, each image is conjoined with genetic and stored experiential information that makes each of us uniquely private. From that complex integral each [of us] constructs at a higher level of perceptual experience . . . his own, very personal, *view from within.*
>
> Mountcastle 1975, p. 131

The menstrual cycle is a normal physiological process unique to females, the experience of which results from a complex interaction of biological and behavioral factors. When a woman becomes seriously symptomatic during any phase of the menstrual cycle, the symptoms must be viewed as a product of the dynamic interaction of all factors.

This assumption is consistent with observations made to the DSM-IV Work Group by some of the group's advisers:

> LLPDD has a phenomenology, no [known] etiology, an uncertain and largely unknown course, responds to a number of nonspecific treatments and a family history that is unclarified. (S. W. Hurt, personal communication, July 1992)

[I]t is a complex weaving of biology, self-perception, interpersonal relationships, and vulnerability to depression. (M. Harrison, personal communication, December 1990)

Clearly, our current nosology is insufficient for classifying this condition. Ideally, we need a multidimensional scheme for classifying all mental disorders that includes developmental appropriateness, internal regulation, contribution of male-female relationships, and extant socioeconomic-cultural supports and stresses. Late luteal phase dysphoric disorder (LLPDD), then, can better serve as "a scientific puzzle which provides a model for sorting out significant crises of conceptualization relevant to the overlap between biomedical and behavioral sciences" (Koeske 1983b, p. 15).

Any attempt to classify LLPDD in DSM-IV will distort the essence of the condition. This does not mean that it should not be classified. It means that the distortion, if it is classified, must be acknowledged. Such a classification, at best, would conceptualize LLPDD as a disturbance of behavioral adaptation. The diagnosis would reflect an imbalance in the dynamic equilibrium between individual, developmental, and socioeconomic forces in a woman's life. In other words, when balance is not reestablished and disturbances in the dynamic equilibrium restrict the developmental process for the woman, a disorder may develop. According to our current understanding of how social change and brain functioning alter each other, the interaction could become internalized as a fixed, self-perpetuating, biologically driven condition. This conceptualization is consistent with the views of others who are proposing an integration model for understanding mental illness (Brown and van Praag 1991; Gabbard 1992; Hartmann 1992; Siever and Davis 1985).

LLPDD as a scientific model allows study from all the perspectives portrayed schematically in Figure 11–1. This schematic representation builds on a basic assumption that women are born with a genetically designed brain and body system that can be influenced and changed by experience and learning. In attempts to study the etiology of LLPDD, one's perspective will differ depending on whether one is viewing the woman's biology, her developmental history, and/or her contemporary circumstances. The latter includes both the woman's internally represented image of her world (i.e., the woman's point of view) and the actual socioeconomic-cultural conditions of her world. All of these loci need study, although the ultimate etiology of LLPDD may rest not in one locus but in the dynamic equilibrium of all loci.

No view can be examined without a definition of LLPDD. The nosological/categorical description of LLPDD in DSM provides this needed definition. The current definition of LLPDD is, however, not fixed. It is the clearest definition we have at the present

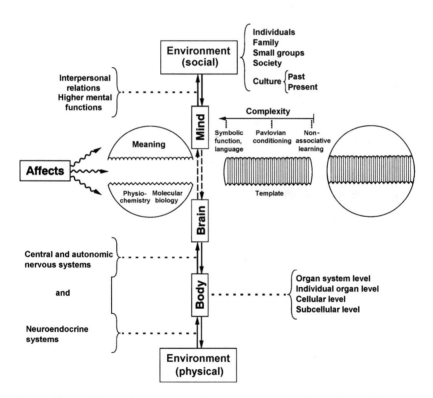

Figure 11–1. Schematic representation of a person in a biopsychosocial environment.
Source. Adapted from Reiser MF: "The Challenge—A Gap Between the Mental and Biological Realms," in *Mind, Brain, and Body.* New York, Basic Books, 1984. Copyright 1984 by Basic Books, Inc. Reprinted by permission of Basic Books, a division of HarperCollins Publishers Inc.

time for a state experienced by a small percentage of women. Our conceptualization of LLPDD is meant to complement the DSM description. We believe that LLPDD requires further research. At the same time, women need treatment for their symptoms and professionals request guidelines for management of symptoms. As research and clinical experience provide more understanding, the definition of the condition and the recommendations for treatment will change.

LLPDD:
Women's Biology and Relationships in the Present

In this book, we have reviewed both empirical issues and sociocultural issues associated with the diagnosis of LLPDD. The first empirical issue addressed is differential diagnosis, presented by Dr. Endicott (Chapter 1). She emphasizes the high prevalence of other psychiatric diagnoses (with symptoms similar or identical to those seen in LLPDD) in women who seek treatment for premenstrual syndrome (PMS). Related to this comorbidity issue, she underscores 1) the difficulty of determining whether a given symptom "occurs" or is "exacerbated" in the luteal phase—some symptoms could occur, whereas others might increase—and 2) the difficulty of determining functional impairment. She also emphasizes that women who do not meet the criteria for the diagnosis of LLPDD because their symptoms are mild or because an ongoing disorder worsens during the luteal phase should not be forgotten.

Drs. Schnurr, Hurt, and Stout (Chapter 2) extend our understanding of Dr. Endicott's points by discussing the consequences of methodological decisions on the diagnosis of LLPDD. They emphasize the fallibility of diagnosis—that clinical diagnosis is not necessarily synonymous with the "true" state or experience of the person, but rather diagnosis is the best guess about the person's state or experience. In other words, the two chapters highlight two sides of the same issue. Dr. Endicott stresses that our current methods offer workable and the best available guidelines for diagnosis;

Dr. Schnurr et al. emphasize that existing methods need further refinement to ensure that the symptoms used to diagnose LLPDD are not chronic symptoms of another condition. In addition, they advise the use of extreme caution in diagnosing LLPDD in women with a current psychiatric disorder. The question could perhaps be raised of whether we should ever diagnose LLPDD in women with mood disorders.

In Chapter 3, Dr. Parry reviews the literature on the biological correlates of PMS. The review is comprehensive and covers the literature through 1991. Readers will feel humbled by learning how much we know and how much we still do not know about LLPDD. Regarding what we do not know, the studies reviewed 1) were predominantly about women with PMS, 2) did not systematically address the issue of comorbidity, and 3) raised the question of whether studies that failed to find an effect are necessarily inconsistent with studies that found an effect. In other words, one study may have found an effect simply because the sample was larger than the study that did not find an effect. Regarding what we do know, Dr. Parry concludes her review with the interesting hypothesis that the most promising area of research about the etiology of affective symptoms in women with LLPDD is the serotonin system.

Dr. Parry's synthesis of what we know about LLPDD is the basis for Chapter 4. Dr. Severino takes Dr. Parry's conclusion about the serotonin system as the focus of a review of the psychiatric literature on serotonin through 1992. She emphasizes that alterations of serotonin regulation seem to be correlated with particular symptoms and behaviors that are found in a number of mental illnesses and are not limited to LLPDD. What Dr. Severino does not do is address whether serotonin's role in regulating mood can account for all symptoms of LLPDD, such as breast tenderness. In addition, she does not address how serotonin's role can be viewed with respect to the roles of the noradrenergic and dopaminergic systems and their influences on emotions and behaviors.

In Chapter 5, Drs. Rivera-Tovar, Pearlstein, and Frank and Ms. Rhodes review the treatment studies of women with PMS. The same difficulties (comorbidity and Type II errors) described for

Dr. Parry's chapter apply to this chapter as well. The chapter includes psychosocial treatment and is comprehensive. The clinician and researcher are cautioned to think through their own approaches to women who seek help for premenstrual complaints.

Dr. Parlee (Chapter 6) raises the question of construct validity (i.e., "external validity") in the diagnosis of LLPDD. In other words, investigators have acted as though the rating scale measures were synonymous with the symptoms they are supposed to measure. In fact, the measures that we rely on to inform us about a woman's daily symptoms are only proxies for her actual experiences, which include personal and social meanings. We must, therefore, constantly remember that the number on the scale is not the same as the symptom in the woman. Dr. Parlee's concern with the meaning of a symptom rating finds a natural extension in the point made by Dr. Schnurr et al. about the fallibility of a diagnosis. Dr. Schnurr's group, however, implies that the way in which rating scales are used is not necessarily a problem. Most parametric statistical tests are robust and not biased when they are used to analyze typical rating scale data. Dr. Parlee's second major contribution, her recommendation of a meta-analysis, arises from the very problems existing in the literature that we delineated, that is, the problems of comorbidity and Type II errors. Such an analysis, then, might compare the effect sizes of two studies that seem to "conflict" because one found a statistically significant effect and the other did not. A meta-analysis would also allow one to examine questions such as 1) the effects of retrospective versus prospective diagnosis and 2) the consistencies between "no difference" versus "differences" in findings.

Dr. Gold's historical chapter (Chapter 7) serves as a bridge between the empirical issues and the sociocultural issues surrounding the diagnosis of LLPDD. She describes the historical framework for the menstrual cycle's relationship to mental illness and to the DSM process. This is followed in Chapter 8 by Dr. Stotland and Ms. Harwood's account of the social, legal, and cultural implications of an LLPDD diagnosis. Here, the primary issue is not methodological problems, but rather the impact of the diagnosis on reifying menstrual disability as a general "given" about women.

Overall, a scholarly approach to this issue is still lacking. Implicit in Stotland and Harwood's chapter is the question of whether there is a causal relationship between the fact that women seek treatment for premenstrual symptoms and the classification of symptoms related to treatment-seeking behavior as illness.

The chapter by Drs. Dan and Monagle (Chapter 9) examines the social and cultural forces that impinge upon women's perception of their psychological and physical state during the premenstrual period. They point out that a society's beliefs about menstruation can influence both expectations about the menstrual cycle and the reporting of symptoms. They urge the need for retrospective and prospective studies from a variety of countries and cultures to further clarify those factors forming sociocultural biases leading to the self-perceptions of women that affect the experience of menstruation. Dr. Severino's commentary (Chapter 10) addresses the role of myths and the diagnosis of LLPDD. The issues she raises demand further discussion and research.

LLPDD: Directions for the Future

Concurrent Concerns

Before addressing recommendations for research on a particular locus, a word must be said about our current diagnostic procedures for LLPDD. We have yet to achieve a consensus on the best tools (e.g., numerical or visual analog scales) and scoring procedures (absolute severity ratings, effect size, etc.; see Chapter 2) for determining symptom change. As one adviser to the DSM-IV Work Group said:

> There is a wide difference across clinicians using LLPDD criteria, which remains undefined quantitatively and heavily dependent on clinician judgment for "severity," amount of premenstrual change, and severity of disruption of daily activities. There is a parallel difference across clinicians using PMS as the term, with some of them producing samples that are more severe in symptomatology and more homogeneous than others using the term LLPDD. I would . . . carry forward with efforts to use terms that

all clinicians can view as useful tools in a consistent diagnosis. (E. W. Freeman, personal communication, February 1992)

In this regard, Dr. Parlee's (Chapter 6) insistence on researchers stringently reporting their procedural details and empirically investigating the impact of their procedures on their results is highly relevant. We must insist on the study of homogeneous, well-defined samples of women and the establishment of better measures of impairment of women's functioning. The issue of reliably differentiating the exacerbation of an existing mental disorder from the coexistence of a mental disorder and LLPDD also needs further attention (see Chapters 1 and 2).

Women's Biology

Much research has been reported regarding the biology of women with premenstrual symptoms (see Chapters 3–5). Yet the methodological problems pertaining to biological studies need further elucidation. In addition, it seems wise to follow the suggestion of Dr. Parlee (Chapter 6) that previous studies of PMS be subjected to a meta-analysis with the goal of resolving some of the apparent disagreements between existing findings.

In addition, our base of normative data across the menstrual cycle needs to be expanded, particularly concerning neuroactive steroids and their relationships to both state and trait phenomena. What occurs biologically during the menstruating years needs to be understood in relation to nonmenstruating states such as prepuberty and menopause, pregnancy, and amenorrheic conditions.

LLPDD, then, needs to be delineated biologically from normative data. A biological indicator for the disorder would be the best means of validating the disorder and a good focus for treatment approaches. In their study, van Praag and colleagues (1991) remind us that psychiatric symptoms are the behavioral expression of a psychological dysfunction, not the dysfunction itself. If LLPDD is a psychological dysfunction, then, we must identify what disturbances of perception, cognition, memory, or information processing in the domains of drive, mood, and hedonic regulation exist and how these correlate with biology.

Since 1987, when LLPDD was formally described in DSM-III-R (American Psychiatric Association 1987), pilot research data have emerged that raise the question of whether women with the disorder differ biologically from women without the disorder. If it exists, the biological difference manifests itself both in measures that differentiate women with LLPDD from women without the condition across the entire menstrual cycle (*trait differences*) and in measures that differentiate women with LLPDD from women without LLPDD with respect to a particular phase of the menstrual cycle (*state measures*). These findings are reviewed in Chapters 3, 4, and 5. Here we would urge that the implicit assumptions of a strictly biological view of these data demand attention. These assumptions have previously been iterated (Koeske 1983a).

The first assumption is that some internal biological difference causes the individual woman's symptoms. Yet, as was pointed out in Chapters 1 and 2, women with LLPDD are inconsistently symptomatic. None of these studies of biological differences considered to what extent mood or behavior produced the physiological measures, although some of them considered the association between the occurrence of the measures. None considered how environmental factors affected the physiological, mood, personality, or behavioral measures. Nor did any of the studies consider how their scoring methods for determining subject selection affected their results.

The second assumption is that "cycle phase is an index of direct biological influence" (Koeske 1983a, p. 6). How do we know, for example, what the meaning of "severe" symptoms is to a woman? How do we know that the "severe" rating is a result of internal physiological changes or of external environmental stresses on the woman? An approach to this issue that might be helpful would be to determine how many times measures of "deviant" serotonin, melatonin, sleep, or temperature parameters are associated with "deviant" premenstrual symptoms in random samples of women.

A Holistic View

To understand the "location" of LLPDD, that is, in the individual or in the social context, the entire system surrounding the woman, in addition to the individual woman, must be studied. Looking at the serotonin system, for example, one would conceptualize how it provides a link to all the state and trait changes seen from the biological view and to changes associated with the behavioral view. The serotonin system has projections to the suprachiasmatic nucleus, which controls circadian rhythms (Moore 1990), and it is excitatory to the paraventricular nucleus, corticotropin-releasing hormone neurons, and the locus ceruleus, which are stress-responsive systems in the central nervous system (Gold et al. 1988). The serotonin system is also associated with thermoregulation (Lesch et al. 1990). (See Chapters 3 and 4 for a review of the research on the serotonin system.)

The effect of serotonin on the suprachiasmatic nucleus might be portrayed as shown in Figure 11–2. According to Linnoila and Virkkunen (1992), concentrations of 5-hydroxyindoleacetic acid (5-HIAA), the end product of serotonin catabolism, in cerebrospinal fluid are strongly affected by season. Levels of 5-HIAA in cere-

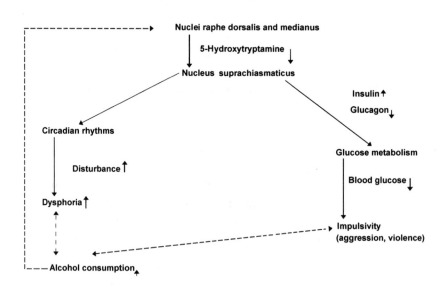

Figure 11–2.   Model of the proposed pathogenesis of impulsivity.
Source. Reprinted from Linnoila VMI, Virkkunen M: "Aggression, Suicidality, and Serotonin." *Journal of Clinical Psychiatry* 53 (Supplement 10):46–51, 1992. Used with permission. Copyright 1992, Physicians Postgraduate Press.

brospinal fluid are lowest in late winter and early spring. Low 5-HIAA concentrations in cerebrospinal fluid are associated with disturbances of day-night activity rhythms and a predisposition to mild hypoglycemia. Indeed, low 5-HIAA concentrations in cerebrospinal fluid are associated with low blood glucose nadirs. Such associations could possibly explain the symptoms related to affect and cognition, as well as sleep and eating behaviors experienced by women with LLPDD, if these measures were found to vary with monthly rhythms of the menstrual cycle in addition to seasonal rhythms.

The effect of serotonin on the corticotropin-releasing hormone and locus ceruleus systems has been described by Gold and colleagues (1988 [Figure 11–3]). Although we cannot yet infer that peripheral serotonin levels predict central serotonergic levels in humans, these relationships have been studied in vervet monkeys, where such a relationship exists (Raleigh and McGuire 1980). Should this apply to humans, given the evidence in Chapter 4 suggesting that women with PMS and LLPDD have decreased binding sites and levels of serotonin in the late luteal phase, this conceptualization could possibly explain the symptoms related to affect and to the autoimmune system.

Studies of nonhuman primates have demonstrated that the serotonin system may also be affected by environmental factors and social interactions (McGuire et al. 1983). In monkeys, serotonin levels are correlated with the monkey's position in the social hierarchy. Male leaders have higher serotonin levels than do male followers, and their serotonin levels fluctuate in response to the behavior of other males:

> [P]hysiologically we may be much more tuned in to the environment than has previously been thought. Different environments create different physiological states, and these, in turn, affect our behavior. (McGuire 1983, p. 77)

Some studies in humans are consistent with the relationship between social status and serotonin reported in monkeys (Hofer 1984; Madsen and McGuire 1984; McGuire 1988). Given these findings, Andrea Rapkin stated:

It is interesting to speculate that the alterations in the hormonal profile triggered by ovulation may for unknown reasons promote post-ovulatory physiological deregulation. Women who are able to regulate this tendency by seeking appropriately rewarding social interactions or "serotonin fixes" may be immune from the symptoms of the PMS. On the other hand, the inability to seek

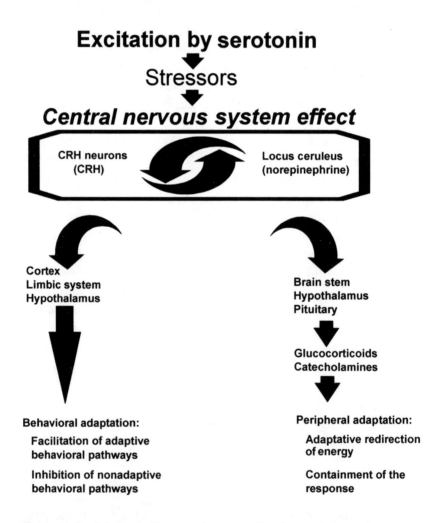

Figure 11–3. Schematic diagram of stress-mediated central effectors. *Source.* Adapted from information appearing in Gold PW, Goodwin FK, Chrousos GP: "Clinical and Biochemical Manifestations of Depression." *New England Journal of Medicine* 319:413–420, 1988. Used with permission.

or receive essential social interactions could lead to further physiologic deregulation and to the manifestation of the symptoms of the PMS. This physiological deregulation may involve a decrease in serotonergic activity. (Rapkin 1992, p. 634)

Women's Developmental History

As noted earlier (Chapter 9), our understanding of women's development is changing. The studies that have approached LLPDD from a behavioral view have suffered from the implicit assumption that LLPDD is nothing more than a social construct that serves psychological, social, political, and legal purposes (Chapter 8). More specifically, studies of LLPDD from a behavioral view constitute a minority of the published literature.

How a woman's biology and environment have interacted over her life span, resulting in her present symptomatology, needs assessment. Under what circumstances does a woman designate an emotional or physical experience a symptom? When, how, and to whom does she describe her distress? What response is she given? How are her relationships affected by a diagnosis of LLPDD (see Chapters 6, 8, and 9)?

The behavioral view would consider how women with LLPDD are similar or different. Do women with LLPDD share similar personality structures, core unresolved conflicts, defense mechanisms for coping, and/or psychosocial situations? The behavioral view would consider how symptoms of LLPDD might be the result of stress due to any psychosocial factor, including cultural and stereotyped myths about women that affect their personal development. Does a particular woman, based on her unique family and developmental experience, attribute a meaning to her experience of the menstrual cycle that engenders stress? A behavioral view would include understanding how the stressful experience of the menstrual cycle is aggravated or ameliorated by the woman's support systems, socioeconomic situation, and group values. More specifically, psychosocial stressors may well be able to affect gene expression, resulting in long-lasting changes in mood, cognition, and behavior (Post 1992). What began as one incident may trigger reactions that become automatic, repetitive (cyclic) experiences. This conceptualization underscores the importance of prevention, that is, preventing first episodes and preventing sensitization.

Here the recommendation of Koeske (1983a) to study the perceptual processes and interpretations used by different women (symptomatic versus asymptomatic), of different ages, life-styles, and life circumstances is relevant. To what extent is LLPDD the symptomatic manifestation of a woman's feeling blocked from acknowledging her experience? She may be blocked by her own views of herself from her past or by "reality's" view of her, given the myths of society. For example, Jean Baker Miller (1986) has described how the assignment of women to the role of caregiver and women's acceptance of this role can lead to symptoms when women have reached the point of not being able to give more, but have not reached the point of feeling allowed to say so. Such a conceptualization would partially explain the emergence of the LLPDD diagnosis at a time in Western society when women are juggling work, home, and children and feeling guilty when unable to do it all.

A conceptualization of LLPDD in the context of a woman's developmental phase has ramifications for treatment, because early interventions may require different treatments than later interventions. Early interventions might include treatments aimed at freeing women from ingrained, painful beliefs about themselves that result in LLPDD symptoms. Later interventions might include treatments aimed at freeing women from the physiological changes that have resulted from altered gene expression that, in turn, continue to reinforce the original ingrained, painful beliefs.

Women's Contemporary Circumstances

Any understanding of a woman's contemporary circumstances will require an understanding both of the internally represented and the practiced elements of her circumstances (Reiss 1989).

Internally represented elements.   An understanding of internally represented elements will draw upon the wisdom of psychology to explain how the woman assimilated her experiences surrounding her family and personal development into an image of what governs social behavior—an image that determines her anticipation of social responses to her behavior. Did the woman's mother have LLPDD? What images of her mother are internalized? What is the influence of a woman's own sex-role stereotyping on her rating of impairment? What does the placebo effect experienced by a woman being treated for LLPDD mean? Of special interest in this regard is the study by Mortola and colleagues (1991), in which eight women with PMS were given a long-acting gonadotropin-releasing hormone agonist to abolish ovarian cyclicity. Once this was accomplished and symptoms improved, a placebo was administered. A reverse placebo effect was reported, in which women experienced the return of their behavioral symptoms despite the fact that ovarian cyclicity was abolished.

Practiced elements.   An understanding of practiced elements will draw upon the wisdom of historians, sociologists, and anthropologists to explain the contemporaneous fit of the woman in her world. How do the woman's cultural and socioeconomic realities and the woman herself mutually influence each other? What is the influence of life cycle changes on the woman's relationships?

In addition, these two perspectives of women's contemporary circumstances need integration. The mechanisms for maintaining the continuity of social behavior over time needs clarification. What first triggers a woman's premenstrual symptoms? How consistent are they? What happens to her symptoms in response to various interventions, such as removal of the woman from some aspect of her environment, treating with medication, and so on? More emphasis is needed on longitudinal studies of women living in a variety of identifiable life-styles:

> [T]his approach would [encourage] delineation of what cycle features (e.g., length, phase duration, presence of ovulation, timing and severity of midcycle, premenstrual and menstrual symptoms, location, intensity and duration of pain, heaviness and duration of menstrual flow, etc.) covary or are mutually exclu-

sive, and what range of differences individual women are capable of experiencing. (Koeske 1983a, p. 14)

Study of these issues is complicated by the fact that much of what we know is unconscious. Any woman is aware of only some of the meanings that determine her symptoms and behavior. We hope, however, that our recommendations for future research will provide avenues for making the unconscious conscious.

References

American Psychiatric Association: Diagnostic and Statistical Manual of Mental Disorders, 3rd Edition, Revised. Washington, DC, American Psychiatric Association, 1987

Brown S-L, van Praag HM (eds): The Role of Serotonin in Psychiatric Disorders. New York, Brunner/Mazel, 1991

Gabbard GO: Psychodynamic psychiatry in the "decade of the brain." Am J Psychiatry 149:991–998, 1992

Gold PW, Goodwin FK, Chrousos GP: Clinical and biochemical manifestations of depression. N Engl J Med 319:413–420, 1988

Hartmann L: Presidential address: reflections on humane values and biopsychosocial integration. Am J Psychiatry 149:1135–1141, 1992

Hofer MA: Relationship as regulators: a psychobiologic perspective on bereavement. Psychosom Med 46:183–197, 1984

Koeske RD: "Curse" is foiled again: thinking clearly about social and psychological factors in the premenstrual syndrome. Paper presented at the annual meeting of the American Psychiatric Association, New York, May 1983a

Koeske RD: The politics of PMS: examining underlying values and assumptions. Paper presented at the American Psychological Association Convention, Anaheim, CA, August 1983b

Lesch KP, Mayer S, Disselkamp-Tietz J, et al: Subsensitivity of the 5-hydroxytryptamine$_{1A}$ (5-HT$_{1A}$) receptor-mediated hypothermic response to ipsapirone in unipolar depression. Life Sci 46:1271–1277, 1990

Linnoila VMI, Virkkunen M: Aggression, suicidality, and serotonin. J Clin Psychiatry 53 (10 [suppl]):46–51, 1992

Madsen D, McGuire MT: Rapid communication whole blood serotonin and the type A behavior pattern. Psychosom Med 46:546–548, 1984

McGuire M: The chemistry of charisma. Science Digest 91:77, 1983

McGuire MT: On the possibility of ethological explanations of psychiatric disorders, in Biological Measures: Their Theoretical and Diagnostic Value in Psychiatry. Edited by Van den Hoofdakker RH. Copenhagen, Denmark, Munksgaard, 1988, pp 7–22

McGuire MT, Raleigh MJ, Johnson C: Social dominance in adult male vervet monkeys: behavior-biochemical relationships. Social Science Information 22:311–328, 1983

Miller JB: Toward a New Psychology of Women. Boston, MA, Beacon Press, 1986

Moore RY: The circadian timing system and the organization of sleep-wake behavior, in Handbook of Sleep Disorders. Edited by Thorpy MJ. New York, Marcel Dekker, 1990, pp 103–115

Mortola JF, Girton L, Fischer U: Successful treatment of severe premenstrual syndrome by combined use of gonadotropin-releasing hormone agonist and estrogen/progestin. J Clin Endocrinol Metab 72:252a–252f, 1991

Mountcastle V: The view from within: pathways to the study of perception. The Johns Hopkins Medical Journal 136:109–131, 1975

Post RM: Transduction of psychosocial stress into the neurobiology of recurrent affective disorder. Am J Psychiatry 149:999–1010, 1992

Raleigh MJ, McGuire MT: Biosocial pharmacology. McLean Hospital Journal 2:73–86, 1980

Rapkin A: The role of serotonin in premenstrual syndrome, in Clinical Obstetrics and Gynecology, Vol 35. Edited by Pitkin RM, Scott JR. Philadelphia, JB Lippincott, 1992, pp 629–636

Reiss D: The represented and practicing family: contrasting visions of family continuity, in Relationship Disturbances in Early Childhood: A Developmental Approach. Edited by Sameroff AJ, Ende RN. New York, Basic Books, 1989, pp 191–220

Siever LJ, Davis KL: Overview: toward a dysregulation hypothesis of depression. Am J Psychiatry 142:1017–1031, 1985

van Praag HM, Brown S-L, Asnis GM, et al: Beyond serotonin: a multiaminergic perspective on abnormal behavior, in The Role of Serotonin in Psychiatric Disorders. Edited by Brown S-L, van Praag HM. New York, Brunner/Mazel, 1991, pp 302–332

✑ Appendix ✑

Terminology in DSM-IV

Since this book was completed, the DSM-IV Task Force has fi-
nalized decisions concerning the content of DSM-IV, and
these recommendations have been approved by the American
Psychiatric Association. As a result of the critical review of the
literature by the Work Group on Late Luteal Phase Dysphoric
Disorder (LLPDD), it was agreed that the studies reviewed support the view that the predominant feature of LLPDD is the
dysphoria that occurs during the premenstrual period. Furthermore, the term *LLPDD* was seen as cumbersome and somewhat
misleading. According to the literature, the symptoms are not
related to the endocrine changes that take place during the late
luteal phase but instead seem to be triggered by them, as
discussed in Chapters 3, 4, and 5, in particular, in this book.
Therefore, the term *premenstrual dysphoric disorder* (PMDD) was
proposed and adopted to replace LLPDD. (See Table 7–2 for criteria for PMDD.)

Recognition is given to the severe and incapacitating dysphoria
that characterizes the disorder by listing PMDD as an example
under "Mood Disorders, Depression, Not Otherwise Specified" in
the main text of DSM-IV. Previously, in DSM-III-R (American Psychiatric Association 1987), LLPDD was listed as an example under
"Unspecified Mental Disorders" in the text. PMDD itself, however,
remains in the appendix of DSM-IV to encourage further research.
It was agreed that the research that has been done to date did not
lead to the inclusion of PMDD in the text as an accepted diagnostic
entity for the reasons discussed in this book.

Reference

American Psychiatric Association: Diagnostic and Statistical Manual of Mental Disorders, 3rd Edition, Revised. Washington, DC, American Psychiatric Association, 1987

ᴣ Index ᴆ

Page numbers printed in **boldface** type refer to tables or figures.